JUST FOR THE
HEALTH
OF IT !   WITH DR. KETCH

Nkechi Olalere (Dr.)

Verbatim Communications
Lagos, Nigeria

Published by Verbatim Communications Limited
+234(0)803 303 6409, 0704 217 8214, 0813 360 2883
Info@verbatimcomms.com
http://www.verbatimcomms.com

JUST FOR THE HEALTH OF IT
ISBN: 978-978-939-802-7

Printed and Bound in Nigeria

Dear reader,

If you are holding this book in your hands, then you most likely believe that healthy living is important. This does not mean that you're perfect; eat all the right things or exercise for the right number of minutes in a day. Neither does it mean that even if you're 'all that'; you no longer need to work at it. Remember that wellness is a journey and not a destination...We have to keep working at it. If you fall off the wagon; dust yourself off, forgive yourself and move on.

The book you have in your hands is actually three books in one.

Book one is on Pregnancy. I feel that pregnant women (especially those experiencing pregnancy for the first time) don't have resources that help them anticipate what's about to happen...especially in our African clime. This book starts the process of addressing these issues and shares with you hilarious things that I did myself on my three 'missionary' journeys.

Book two is on Parenting. Trust me, I do not claim to be an expert but I hope that by sharing my experience, you're better equipped to handle your children.

Book three is on diet, exercise and so much more. This is mainly a collection of questions people have asked me over time and posts that I had made on my blog concerning the issues highlighted. If you've ever wondered whether there's a magic pill for weight loss, you'll love this part.

All in all, I hope that y'all; singles, married, young ones, grandparents, men and women of all colours and races will find something useful in this book.

I'd love to hear your comments after reading and of course, learn what you would like me to address in future parts of these different books.

You can reach me on healthylivingwithdrketch@gmail.com, www.facebook.com / healthylivingwithdrketch, www.chatwithdrketch.com and finally follow me on Twitter @ketchilola

ACKNOWLEDGMENT

My life has gone down various paths in my journey of life and at the beginning of each path, many, including myself, have been left confused and dumbfounded...almost 😊

I would like to thank God Almighty...the ONE who has made it possible for me to remain true to myself and my passion...and smile while running down the many paths that have called to me.

My children;
Bolaji, my conscience, who keeps me on the straight and narrow. Chidera, 'MojaDera,' who continues to teach me about patience. Fisoye, my genius...who keeps reminding me what all that patience I'm learning is for. Thank you all for teaching me so much and bearing with me as I learn about parenting by parenting y'all. 😊
Thanks for all the subtle and not so subtle 'jabs' which have added character to this book.

My mother, Dr Pauline Onyekonwu, one of the most hardworking women I've ever known. Thanks for standing by me, believing in me and pushing me to do greater things.

My sister, Nonye Okonkwo; quiet but strong. Thanks for being my constant sounding board for ideas, bright and sometimes, not so bright 😊

My Pastor, Pius Isiekwena; you have been a blessing to me...encouraging me and checking up on me and indeed pushing me to write this book.

My Social Media family, (Facebook, Twitter and blog) for confirming to me every single day, that my chosen path meets a deep need in you.

So many people, too numerous to mention, who have played one part or the other in shaping me into the person I have become and have been part of my story.

Finally, I acknowledge all the obstacles and challenges, human and material, which I have encountered in my life journey. Y'all made me stronger and indeed, confirmed what the Bible said that, 'when men are cast down, then thou shalt say, there's a lifting up.'

May God, reward all your labours of love and grant you all your hearts' desires.

Nkechi Olalere
2014

DEDICATION

I dedicate this book to Boccifi.
You make my world beautiful.

PREGNANT?
Don't Be Ignorant!

TABLE OF CONTENTS

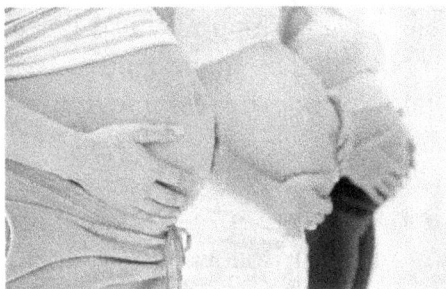

Introduction

...In the beginning

Pregnancy is such a precious time. I will go so far as to say, it is an amazing time; the beginning of life. I can just see the faces of all of you who spent the entire nine months of pregnancy in hospital beds or vomiting or just feeling 'horrible.' I get it! It also wasn't all fun and games for me during any of my three 'pilgrimages.' But this is one situation where the end justifies the means because the thought of how the situation would end, should make up for all the discomfort...I hope.

How many of us come prepared? None of us, really. We just roll with the punches and pray we come out tops.

I am a doctor, but even with all that medical information, I was not prepared for what my body threw up at me when I got pregnant. Over time, especially ever since our wellness television programme, 'Tips For Healthy Living with Dr Ketch' started, I have had more pregnant women ask questions that clearly show how 'starved' they are for information. And so, the idea for this book was born. It's a collection of my recollections of my pregnancies, peppered with some of your questions, written in simple everyday language that we can all relate with…all of it valuable information that I believe is important for every new mum. I hope that by sharing my own experiences, you will feel equipped to handle yours by learning from some of my hilarious mistakes.

Enjoy the read and please drop me a line with questions or your thoughts on any of the following: www.chatwithdrketch.com, @ketchilola. www.facebook.com/healthylivingwithdrketch

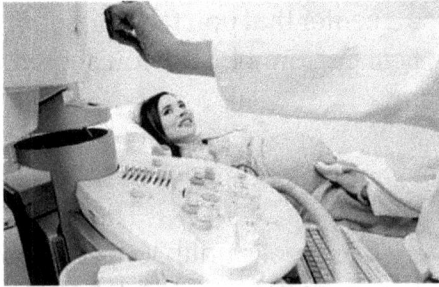

Before Birth

ANC, Haematinics et al

Did you find yourself wondering what time to register for antenatal care (ANC)? If this is your first pregnancy, then you're probably more worried than most. But the practical truth is that you should register for Antenatal care as soon as you realize you are pregnant.

To prepare for that visit, you should remember the date of your last menstrual period, past medical history and immunisations as well as infections you have had in the past such as Chicken Pox. Also check your family history for medical problems such as high blood pressure, diabetes, child-birth abnormality, sickle cell disease and other illnesses. Be generous with information about any and everything that may affect your baby's health such as lifestyle habits like smoking and alcohol drinking.

Ultrasound scan will be carried out to check whether your baby is in the right place, the number of babies you are pregnant with and the age of your pregnancy. Other screening tests will also be carried out on your urine and blood, to confirm your blood level, blood group, genotype, infections such as syphylis and Hepatitis B. HIV screening may also be done after counselling, if you give consent.

You should choose a center that you feel confident with as regards the quality of the medical personnel, and you should freely discuss your birth plan with them.

In the first instance, antenatal care will be scheduled once every four weeks until the pregnancy is 28 weeks. Thereafter, the appointments are scheduled every two weeks until 36 weeks and thereafter, every week till delivery. This is the normal schedule, but your care giver may decide to assign you shorter appointments if there are other factors to be considered like the presence of hypertension in pregnancy or indeed to review results of tests you had been sent to do.

As for those drugs that you are given with, if you're like me and hate to take drugs, then this is a big deal! 😊   But you do have to take them. The most crucial period is within the first four weeks of conception, i.e. about six weeks from the first day of your last period.

The folic acid you will be asked to take ensures that your baby does not end up with abnormalities of the spine and also helps build up your red blood cells in combination with the other drugs given. You've got to be religiously committed to taking these drugs to give your pregnancy the greatest chance of a good outcome. Therefore, start taking the right doses of folic acid as soon as you start considering getting pregnant or as soon as you test positive for pregnancy.

So, have you taken today's dose? Let's go do it now. 😊

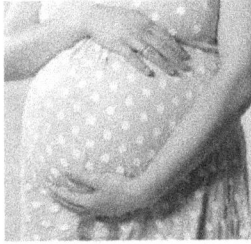

'Baby in the tummy; its all up to mummy...is it?

Do you remember your first pregnancy? This question is directed at the ladies (obviously ☻). We know how all the pains and stress of pregnancy melted away once we held our babies. I remember mine very vividly.

To start with, I had no idea I was pregnant. I was doing my medical internship then, and I worked in the Emergency Room (ER). This particular ER was extremely busy, most of the times and specifically at this period in question. So, I couldn't afford the distraction of a fever...because that was what I kept experiencing with, fever and that peculiar Nigerian symptom of internal heat. ☺ I shrugged it off and kept going. But these symptoms were going nowhere! They worsened such that when I smelt perfume, I would throw up and I had this absolutely disgusting taste in my mouth. Sounds like malaria, yes? Well, I freely confess to not being the best patient and so I didn't run a test neither did I treat myself. I just figured it would go away.

Quick disclaimer: please don't practice this when you are pregnant or at any time at all.

Anyways, matters came to a head when I practically shut down my kitchen. I couldn't stand the smell in there. My kitchen was filled with lots of essences for baking: vanilla, strawberry, banana, orange, etc. The mix of the essences was just not agreeing with my nose. Every time I went in there, I headed straight to the bathroom to vomit. And the bathroom? That was no help either. The detergent I was using at that time suddenly became nauseating to me. Well, I felt I could do without cooking and shut down my kitchen, but hey, I had business to transact in my bathroom every day and so something had to give!

I got rid of the detergent and had to switch to something else. And finally, some part of my medically trained brain asked the question, 'are you pregnant?' I was in shock! My husband was in Port Harcourt while I was rounding off my internship. I didn't quite plan for dealing with this on my own and so I sorta prayed for this cup to pass me by…at least for the moment.

It was at that moment that I decided to go get those symptoms checked out. As I already had it in my head that I was pregnant, I decided to go do a scan to confirm this…not the most orthodox way of confirming pregnancy I know. 😊   And, yes, I found out that I was pregnant! The rest, as they say, is history!

This is one of the reasons why I always empathise when I watch TV shows that tell us how some women were far along before they knew they were pregnant. The ones that actually put to bed before they knew they were pregnant stretch the imagination but may not be far-fetched. For a first time mother, this is particularly important as she may not know what signs to look out for, what's normal and what's not. Putting it in context… I am a medical doctor, and I didn't even know I was pregnant. 😊

This is about the glorious state of pregnancy, the normal signs and the red flags. The red flags are the signs that may spell trouble and which should be checked out immediately without waiting for the next pre-natal (antenatal) clinic visit.

We'll start with the normal:

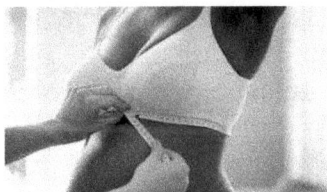

Breast tenderness: This is inevitable as your breast ducts prepare for the job of lactation. Bra sizes could go up from 1 to several sizes up. Be sure to get a good support bra and keep going up sizes as your breast size increases. This will help reduce sagging.

Vaginal Discharge: A thin milky discharge is normal during pregnancy.

Heart burn and Constipation: These happen due to one of the hormones produced during pregnancy. The antenatal supplements, especially those containing high doses of iron may worsen the heart burn and also play a part in worsening constipation, therefore, use them judiciously in consultation with your caregiver.

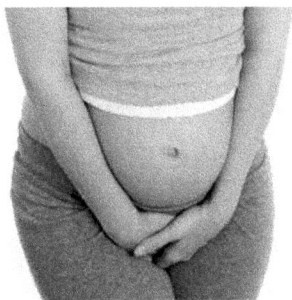

Frequency of urination: As the baby grows in the uterus, it presses on the bladder making you feel like urinating more often. Early in the pregnancy before your tummy even begins to show, you may experience this symptom due to an increase in blood flowing to your kidneys. Always mention it to your caregiver so that they can distinguish it from bladder infections.

Tiredness: As your body works overtime to support a growing life inside you, you would feel exhausted.

Food cravings and aversions: Well, I certainly had loads of aversions with my first pregnancy. I can't remember any cravings as I couldn't get any food to stay down. However, some people develop a craving for the oddest, craziest foods when pregnant. Go easy on eating for two though...the healthy living dictum of eating loads of fruits or vegetables and low calories does not change during pregnancy. The more you gorge or give in to the food cravings, the more work you have to do to get it off after giving birth to the baby. However, if you find yourself craving things like clay and sand, please see your doctor as it could be a sign of iron-deficiency anaemia.

Morning sickness or nausea

This is due to the hormones of pregnancy (again!). This may be mild or so severe that the person actually gets hospitalized. If your nausea is severe, please see your doctor. But generally, you can help push this back by eating some bland food especially in the mornings when it is worse like crackers or cheese. I, personally, preferred tangy tastes and so tangy (sour-tasting candies etc) were a favourite for me. Not very healthy, I know 😊

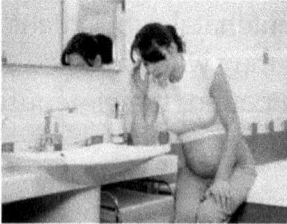

Now for the red flags...these have to be heard and checked out by your obstetrician immediately.

Significant bleeding: Once you spot any sign of bleeding, notify your doctor and let them decide if it's a problem. Better safe than sorry.

Crampy abdominal pain: Pain experienced in your abdominal

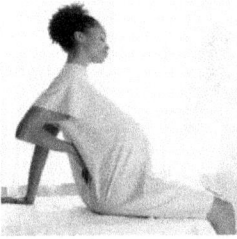

region, i.e. the lower part of your tummy, could be a sign of a threatened miscarriage.

Severe nausea/vomiting: This could lead to dehydration which could affect the baby adversely.

Too little weight gain or too much weight gain: Try to keep weight gain between 8 to 16kg during the pregnancy. Your doctor could have recommended more or less depending on your pre-pregnancy state.

Pain or burning sensation when urinating: This could be a urinary tract infection. It needs to be dealt with.

Vaginal discharge: Foul smelling, yellow or greenish colour could indicate an infection and could affect your baby.

High fever: This could signify an infection.

So ladies, enjoy this fabulous state of pregnancy. Guys, give them all the support they need...and deserve. By the way, did I forget the amazing mood swings that are a very normal part of this state? Guys, be sure to respect and lovingly manage that. It's all those hormones running amok in the body. You play a huge role in ensuring a successful outcome of the pregnancy.

As for me, I'm done with all that stuff. I'm a grandmother in waiting! Loads of years before we get there, though! Keep healthy people and don't let pregnancy get you down. It's really not a sickness And the products of this process live forever in our hearts.

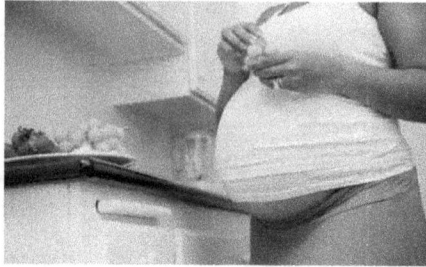

Eating for Two?

I'm sure everyone has heard the 'eating for two' fable. It is indeed, an old wives' tale because if you were eating for two, the assumption would probably be that you should double your calorie requirement for a day....so for a woman that probably means you can get away with taking in as much as four thousand calories per day!!! That's a recipe for disaster.

Pregnancy is associated with increased cravings and of course growth of the baby, but you do not need significantly more calories to cope with this state. The recommended weight gain for pregnancy is eight to sixteen kilograms in all (with an average of twelve kilograms).

Let me break it down for you.

During your first trimester, you actually do not need more calories than when you were not pregnant. You can continue with the activities you used to do before, including exercise. However, exercise should be toned down from vigorous to moderate.

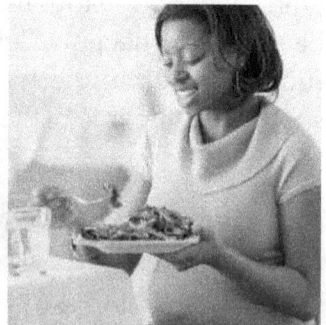

[Moderate exercise is any physical activity that you perform and you're still able to carry on a conversation without running out of breath…that's as simple an explanation as it goes.   It includes walking, swimming, dancing, pregnancy exercises - these are taught in some antenatal classes- stretching and relaxation exercises. Remember that you must never start on any exercise regimen without discussing with your doctor who knows your specific medical history.]

Please note that you should never exercise to the point of exhaustion, do not over-heat yourself and this is not the time to engage in activities that make you jump…partly because you are prone to injuries of the ligaments (like sprains)and because, it's just not safe at the time. I always used to know I was pregnant whenever I sprained my ankle…it happened in two out of three pregnancies! It may not be an exact science, but it worked for me.   (Just kidding…don't try this at home)

During your second trimester, your calorie needs start to increase. The recommended increase in calorie intake is about three hundred calories per day over the pregnancy requirements. Does this sound like much? It actually is not! A popular brand of wheat biscuits with a serving size of four is two hundred and forty calories. That's wheat biscuit).   So, imagine the quantum of calories in the other junk foods we crave for during this period! Take the time to read labels of food packs and check what the serving size is. If there are two serving portions in a tub of ice cream and you finish the whole tub, you've clearly eaten double the calories that are written on the tub!

In the final trimester, the calorie requirement increases some more to about 400 calories per day over the pre-pregnancy levels per day. Note that for multiple pregnancies (twins, triplets etc.), the calorie needs are an extra 400 calories in the second trimester and an extra five hundred to six hundred calories in the third trimester.

With all these rules, are you now wondering what to eat? It's essentially the same things you did before you got pregnant…assuming you were eating right. 🙂 More fruits, veggies and complex carbohydrates which are rich in fibre and keep you feeling full for a longer period of time. Some examples of complex carbohydrates include beans, oatmeal, sweet potatoes, brown rice, etc. Load up on proteins too (fish, chicken, etc.) and calcium-rich foods like yoghurt, skimmed milk…you don't want to experience those muscle cramps of pregnancy. They can be excruciating! I know…I've had them. 🙂

Eat 5 small meals a day: breakfast, snack, lunch, snack and dinner. This should keep the hunger pangs at bay and deal with the cravings. You probably will still crave stuff: Iyaalamala's food, ice cream with all the toppings or a 'ginormous' (for the uninitiated, this is a word formed from a mixture of gigantic and enormous. Cute, right?) burger. And guess what? You can give in once in a blue-moon, just don't make it a habit!

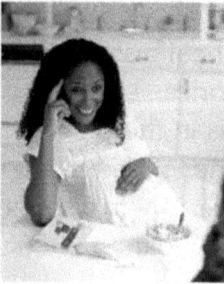

If you take in more calories than you need, you run the risk of having a big baby with all the complications associated with that during pregnancy and delivery and of course, it's harder to get back to your pre-pregnancy weight after the baby. A study has also shown that babies fed junk food while the womb develop a taste for it and may become junk food addicts later. You don't want to do that to your baby, I 'm sure.

Help! I'm pregnant, and my doctor says my baby is big!

Just in case you weren't quite convinced by the 'you don't have to eat for two' advice, this question on big babies should help.

Q: I am an expectant mother in the last trimester. My doctor told me my baby is big. What does this mean? Am I safe?

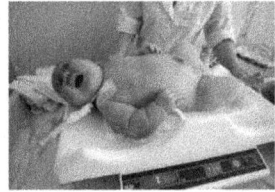

A: The focus should be on what caused the big baby and what can be done to ensure that you and baby come out okay.

Big babies are usually seen in women who:
- Are diabetic prior to pregnancy.
- Have gestational Diabetes (Diabetes that is observed during pregnancy).
- Are obese.
- Have had another big baby before.
- Have had a lot of babies (from the fifth pregnancy, the risk of big babies increases).
- Have excessive weight gain during pregnancy.
- Are older. From age 35 years, the risk of having a big baby increases.
- Have pregnancies that are overdue. When a pregnancy is more than 2 weeks overdue, the chances of a big baby are increased.

For women with big babies (fetal macrosomia) a vaginal delivery may not be a complete no no! However, your OBGYN will weigh the risk of that against your medical history and other pre-existing medical conditions. Potential complications include having genital tract tears during delivery, prolonged labour and rupture of the uterus. The babies may be born with a higher than normal blood sugar level and be prone to childhood obesity.

However, none of this needs to happen if you are registered in a good centre under the care of a qualified obstetrician. In these centres, all possible complications are anticipated during pregnancy and at the time of delivery.

To prevent this, remember that feeding for two is a fable. You don't really need to eat like a horse 😊 you and your baby don't need that much food (an average of 12kg weight gain for nine months...a little over 1kg per month!) include some exercise-gentle stretches and walks, with your doctor's knowledge and advice - and be sure that Diabetes is controlled, if you had this before pregnancy.

For the remainder of your pregnancy, be sure to follow your doctor's instruction on weight gain, medications and other health safety measures to the letter! Let's share the good news when the baby is born.

All the best!

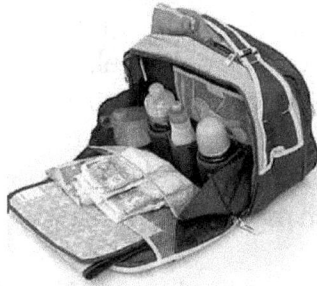

ALL PACKED UP AND READY TO GO?

Is your hospital bag ready? I use the word 'bag' advisedly!
I know some of you have huge bags...scratch that! I know some of you have huge boxes packed full with every imaginable (and unimaginable) thing you can think of. But guess what? You just may not need all those. Are you also worried about what to expect, how much the pain would be? Well, you should certainly read this.

As a medical student and young doctor, I spent a lot of time in the labour wards and seeing women in labour gave me very clear ideas about what I wanted and did not want to happen when it was my turn. First, all that screaming and moaning and shouting at any and everybody, including present or absent husbands who got them pregnant, was not for me! Nope, I wasn't going to do that I was going to maintain my dignity and if need be, just moan fashionably. I had also been told that a popular old wives' tale had it that if you screamed in your first pregnancy, you were likely to scream for every other pregnancy afterwards. Seriously!!! Of course, I knew there was no truth to that, but not screaming was also in keeping with my original plan, so why not?! The funniest part of this plan is the fact that I had no plan to use epidural anaesthetic - the injection that makes women not feel pain during child birth! So how on earth was I not going to scream? Not the best of plans, aye!?!

Then, all that drama with the pregnant women practically stripping themselves naked from the pain et al.- that just wasn't going to be me! Nope! I would check into the hospital with my fashionable 'big gown,' red in colour…of course…to suit the purpose. Stripping naked in front of all those male doctors was certainly not for me…most of them I knew, making it even more embarrassing!

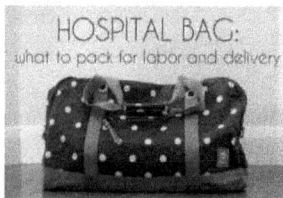

HOSPITAL BAG:
what to pack for labor and delivery

My hospital bag? Oh, I felt I had time. And so, it was two days before I eventually gave birth that I finally felt the pressure to ensure that I was all packed up. After I had come back from shopping, I went into labour the next day and put to bed early hours of the day after. You don't want that to be you!

Let's make this easier. Here are the top essentials for your carry-on luggage to the hospital

We'll break it up into things for you, things for him (your loving hubby) and things for your new baby. We'll further break the requirements for mum and baby into 'need to have,' 'nice to have' and 'absolutely not'!

Things for mum

Need to have:
- Health Insurance or plan card: You don't want to have to pay money when you're on a plan that covers this service
- Tooth paste or brush, creams and lotions and other toiletries including make-up: Yes, make-up. We still have to look and smell good through it all.
- Hair brush or comb

- A robe or wrapper
- Maxi Sanitary towels
- Undergarments (nursing bras and panties…no thongs. Trust me, those maxi pads were not designed for thongs)
- Night gown
- Slippers
- Non-skid socks: For those moments when you have to walk up and down the hospital corridor before the event.
- Scrunchies and hair bands to hold up your hair
- Snacks (healthy options of course) to nibble on afterwards if it's too late for hospital kitchen to serve up something. If the hospital has a vending machine, this may not be necessary as you will be able to get some quick snacks from there.

Nice to have:
- Camera with charger and other consumables needed
- Baby book
- Mobile phone and charger
- Recharge cards or airtime for your phone to notify people when it's over
- A 'wow' outfit to go home in. Honestly, this is a must-have for me now that I'm older and wiser. 😊 I didn't have it any of the three times I passed through it, though, but I should have. 😊 Truth is, you can very well go home in the outfit you came to the hospital in except you're the princess of Wales, and you know the whole world will be waiting outside to see what you look like.
- Ipod/mp3 with your favourite tunes: This helps you pass the time in between contractions when you're waiting.

- Wine to celebrate with: What better way to welcome baby into the world?! ☺
- Bath towel: The hospital will certainly have their supply of these but if you're picky, please bring yours along.
- Your favourite pillow and coloured pillow cases to differentiate from the hospital bed linen.

For him
- Tooth paste/brush and toiletries
- Change of clothes
- Snacks (healthy ones) for him

For baby
Need to Have
- First wears
- Car seat
- Shawl and other outdoor clothes
- Change of clothes

Absolutely Not

A year's supply of clothes for baby 😷
For those of us in Nigeria and perhaps other parts of Africa, there are some other essentials:
- Olive oils
- Cotton wool
- Methylated spirit
- Cord clamp

And just in case you are wondering about all those fancy plans I made about not screaming and being fashionable, I'll enlighten you.

I started off just moaning…as fashionably as I could. Then I graduated to hitting the bedside locker instead of screaming, and I pretty much kept it that way for the whole period. Then the gown…I did get to wear it. However, by no stretch of imagination can I suggest that I was ladylike through it all. I certainly bared it all…and several times too! How on earth can you manage to keep it all together when you have to open up your legs every now and again for the cervical dilatation (how many centimetres dilated you are) to be checked? Hardly likely. So, in retrospect, I advise you to go with the flow. The doctors have absolutely no desire to make you feel uncomfortable and will preserve your modesty as much as practicable. Oh and, by the way, I also hated the back rubs! They just exacerbated the pain for me.

As a footnote, when I was having my last baby (my third), I screamed like a banshee. Methinks it was all that pent-up emotion from the first two births that I didn't quite release. I went to town. You could hear my voice from nine blocks away…I'm certain of this!

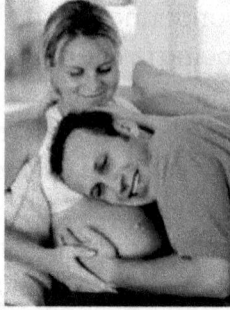

SOMETHING FOR DADDY

Fathers are so significant in the scheme of things that it's well worthwhile to include a page or more on him, his roles and what he's going through at this time.

How do I cope with my 'new' wife?!

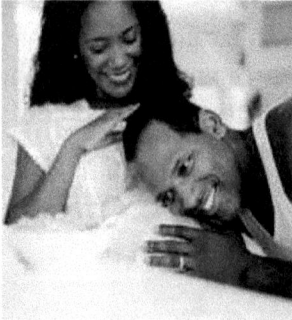

Pregnancies affect daddies too! First, this amazing woman they love suddenly becomes a bundle of emotions. He's not sure from day to day, what is appropriate. Today, he wasn't affectionate enough; tomorrow, he's too affectionate in front of people? And why does she keep bursting into tears at the most improbable time? What's going on? Is this the picture of marriage he has to deal with for the rest of his life from now?

"And then, there's the constant chatter about the baby! Honestly, I get it. I'm excited too. This is our first baby. A symbol of our love for the whole world to see. I truly can't wait also to see whether he or she will look like me or her (honestly, I don't even care!) or whether he or she will share those character traits from my family that have been strong through a lot of generations. But honestly, I don't want to spend every waking moment talking about that nor picking out clothes, colours, etc. I sincerely want to be there for my wifey but this is just too much. Am I being selfish?"

No, you're not! It's a normal reaction which you're entitled to, but really have to deal with quickly. That didn't sound very sympathetic, right?

Some of the issues on the minds of fathers are worries over an 'impending' starvation of sexual intimacy, increase in financial responsibilities and so on. These are enough to stress the potential Daddy out and lead to the release of the stress hormone, Cortisol, which reduces libido. But, pregnancy does not mean starvation of any kind. Provided your wife's obstetrician has not noted any situation that makes sexual intimacy a 'problem, ' you and your wife are at liberty to continue with your pre-pregnancy routine. In fact, some women actually have more of a libido while pregnant than at other times. Now you do have to commit to 'earnestly' praying for your wife to fall into this category.

Hey, but guess what? Nature gives you nine months to prepare financially, emotionally and otherwise for the very demanding role of being a father and an even more caring husband- emphasis on the 'more.' You do need to be a tower of strength for your wife who's probably going through pregnancy for the first time. Even if it's not the first time, those hormones truly don't care. They are at work promptly everyday ensuring your wife feels emotionally 'on fire' just as much as the first time!

And please plan to be around for your baby's birth. It really helps your wife go through it all knowing that you are there looking out for her and helping her through the pain. The stories of fathers who love their wives even more after they see them go through the very painful process of labour is also a great incentive for the ladies to want their men there. We can all take some more love...that can't be too much

Just remember through it all that these too, shall pass. The whole drama of pregnancy with all its shenanigans will most definitely blow over and you get to have your beautiful wife all to yourself again...errrrm with one significant addition! Only a matter of time.

Daddy or Father...which do you plan to be?

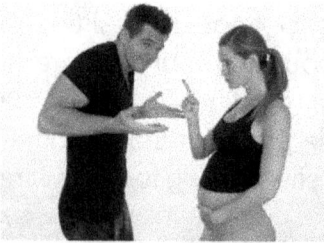

Whenever, it's Fathers' day, people roll out drums to celebrate fathers, dead or alive. Mine, unfortunately is dead...but the memories linger on (sigh!)

Methinks that these are moments for sober reflection. So, for would-be fathers, the question is, 'am I going to be a father or a daddy?' Now before I start with my definitions, let me quickly issue the disclaimer that the definitions I am about to give probably do not exist in any other dictionary available as at today or planned for the future, except 'the Dr Ketch book of stuff and things' (copyright reserved). There! That's done. On to the business of the day!

As I was going to say, a father is...well, one who fathers a child. In other words he provides the counterpart chromosome for a baby to be made. A bit like counterpart funding for a project. This doesn't require much in terms of time, emotion, focus, etc. Anyone can do this. This man is not invested in any way in his children's lives: financially, emotionally, physically, socially and mentally. He's an occasional father! He probably presents the children for photo opportunities whenever he feels it looks good and can give him a leg up, if you get what I mean.

But then, there's daddy! Daddy is a special being! He's the one who sees mummy through the pregnancy and ensures she's physically and emotionally healthy by ensuring she attends antenatal classes, takes her ANC drugs and reduces her work burden. Daddy, it is who stands by mummy when the labour pains come and she has to get to the hospital. Daddy, it is who stands by mum when it is time to push and practically pushes with her until the precious bundle of joy is birthed. Remember the change of clothes for him? It's because we presume that Daddy will be spending the night pacing the floor or carrying out back rubbing duties.

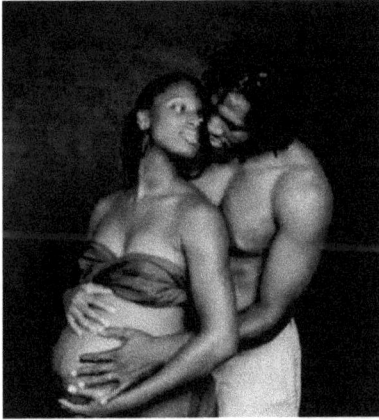

From this time, daddy plays an even more active role: changing diapers, playing and bonding with baby, attending PTA meetings, concerts and recitals even when all that is on offer is a cacophony of screeching voices (if you get what I mean). In fact, daddy would get up and say, 'that's my baby over there' with such pride that people would look and shake their heads with a mixture of pity – at the thought that he finds anything sonorous about the voices he is hearing - and amusement at his very clearly evident love! Daddy will attend these events, re-scheduling meetings just so he can be there and openly chastise other 'very-busy-I-am-very-important-and-don't-have-time-for-these-events' fathers for not doing so! Is it any wonder that the children grow up, socially, emotionally and mentally healthy knowing the exact role model needed for life and the choices they have to make when it's their turn?

So where would you like to fall in? Daddy or father? You can make a choice today. Thereafter, history will be the judge!

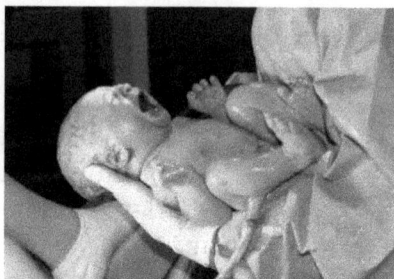

After Birth

Taking your baby home.   What next?

Remember the baby book I mentioned earlier? Be sure not to forget it, or you may pay dearly for it. I'll share my story with you.

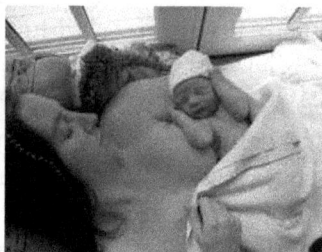

When I had my first baby, of course, I had a baby book and took loads of pictures and filled up the baby book. There was hardly any empty page. I had the first lock of hair clipped, I had the outline of the foot drawn, I had the first picture with her face all wrinkled up in there.

By the time I had my second baby, I was a bit more blasé…been there, done that, if you get what I mean So, the pictures were fewer, the moments captured less and events recorded fewer too.

With my last baby, it was absolutely horrible. I didn't buy the baby book and could not, for the life of me, remember to take pictures of my baby. This really was a difficult time in my life, so perhaps, that's a good excuse but guess what? When the day comes, that explanation will not suffice. And that day came!

Every so often, my daughters would bring out their baby books and we would reminisce about events from their childhood. At these times, my son would ask me about his own book and about anecdotes from his childhood too. This started off without incident and I managed to smooth over awkward moments until the time when this could no longer work. My son started asking pointed questions about his baby book, about events backed up by pictures etc. I could see the look of 'I'm not quite sure she loves me. How come she made all this effort for my sisters and not for me?' And so that settled it! I started the project with my second daughter.

We brought out our big bag of pictures and got to work bringing out all my son's pictures that ever existed. I then bought the biggest baby book that ever existed and we set to work pasting all the pictures therein. It was a labour of love and despite a couple of gaps...like trace of hands and feet at certain ages, it still looked amazing when we were done, even if I say so myself! So, don't get yourself into this mess, be armed with your baby book and make sure all those life events are well represented, starting with your baby's first picture when you get home.

Now that you're home, if you live anywhere in Africa, be ready for the deluge of visitors. They all mean well, but not all of them will observe the basic rules of hygiene needed to keep a baby safe. Imagine this scenario: an elderly woman hurrying back from the market to come to your house to see your new baby. She quickly makes a beeline for the baby cot in the corner of the room to pick up your baby with those unwashed germy hands that have touched all sorts all day! How do you tell this kind-hearted Mama or Iya Sikira that you'd want her to wash her hands or better still just leave the baby for now? And what about you, what's right to do

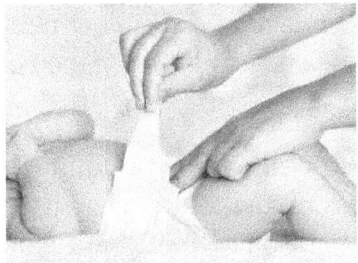

and what's not? Let's give you some pointers.

- As much as is practicable, wash your hands before picking up your baby. This ensures that you're not transferring germs from the outdoors or anywhere else you're coming from to the baby.
- Wash your hands after a diaper change. This should be done routinely after every diaper change be it that your baby urinated or pooed. This ensures that you are not transferring germs from your baby's diapers to food or even other people when you pat, hug or dress them after a diaper change.
- Encourage visitors to wash their hands before picking up the baby. You can keep a bottle of sanitizer by the side to encourage this hygienic practice if hand washing is not practicable at that time.
- Keep a flannel on your shoulder when you carry your baby on your shoulder. You know how children love to suck every surface that comes in contact with their lips. Well, don't let that surface be your shoulder. Imagine all the germs and bacteria that have been deposited there all day. You don't want them to end up in your baby's tummy.
- Pack and disinfect baby's rattles and toys at least once a day to ensure that when they play with them, they are clean.

Spend time bonding with the baby. This is not just for mummies…daddies also need to bond with the babies and get the baby off to a great, emotionally sound start in life.

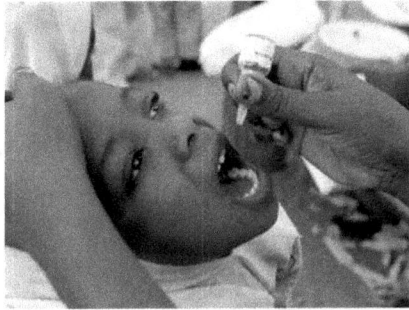

Immunization 101

In a country like Nigeria, the burden of disease is made worse by the fact that some of these diseases are vaccine-preventable. The National Program on Immunization(NPI) in Nigeria has delineated specific diseases that children have to be inoculated against from birth. There are a couple of extra vaccines that paediatricians also advice children to have. I have been asked whether they are necessary since they do not appear on the NPI schedule. Well, put it this way, cost is always an issue in making drugs or any product or service available for the whole population. Some other vaccines are in the works and will be made available to everyone soon. In the meantime, focus on the compulsory ones and if you can afford it, certainly add on the extras until they become available and free of charge. Let's give you a quick reminder class, about the vaccines that your child should get.

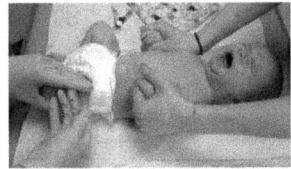

- At birth, BCG and Hepatitis B vaccines are given. The former protects against tuberculosis, which, unfortunately, is making a comeback with the advent of HIV/AIDS. At six, ten and fourteen weeks, the Oral Polio Vaccine

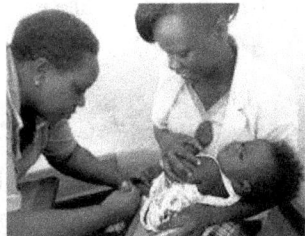

- (OPV) and the pentavalent vaccines are due.
- The pentavalent vaccines include those for DPT (Diphtheria, Pertussis and Tuberculosis), Hepatitis B and Haemophilus Influenza. Booster doses for OPV are due at 18 months, 4-6 years and 10 years. Booster doses for DPT are due at 18 months and 4-6 years. Hepatitis B can cause long term complications of the liver (cirrhosis) if contracted. A booster dose is to be given at 5 years. Hepatitis B vaccine can also be taken in adulthood especially for people who are at risk; five doses are required.
- At nine months, the measles and yellow fever vaccines are due. A booster dose for yellow fever is required once in every ten years.

The above are the compulsory ones required for every child by the NPI.

- Before the age of nine months, an additional vaccine that could be given is the Rotavirus vaccine. It appears that even hand washing does not protect against this virus. Two doses of this vaccine are usually given before the age of 6 months at one month interval.

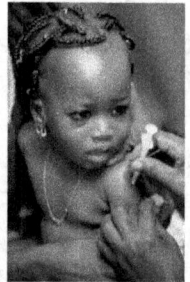

- Other vaccines that could be given include chicken pox vaccine (from one year of age), pneumococcal vaccines (at 2, 4 and 13 months of age), and typhoid vaccines (with boosters every three years).

Evidently, the issue has been laid to rest. The NPI vaccines are critical and every child should get them. Let's give our under 5's survival rates a major boost.

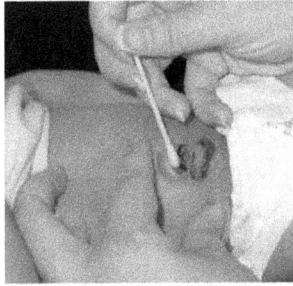

Cord Care, Sitz Bath et al

Do you remember trying to sit down after you delivered your baby? If you had an episiotomy (a surgical tear to help ease the passage of the baby), you probably froze in shock at the pain, right? Well, I did. It was just plain excruciating to attempt to sit, much less, adjust yourself to a more comfortable sitting position. Then, do you remember the first time after that when you tried to pass gas? It was sheer agony! Agony that melts away as you behold the bundle of joy that was a result of that process. Now, if you haven't had your baby yet, this may sound very scary, but there's a solution for this pain.

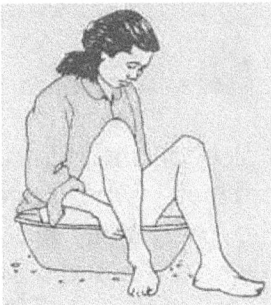

Ever heard of a Sitz bath? It's a warm water bath that helps cleanse the perineum. Just in case you wondered, the perineum is the space between the rectum and the genitals. The right temperature is the one that you can handle without sustaining burns. Putting a few drops of this water on the inner surface of your wrist can help confirm this.

Plain warm water is sufficient, but some people add salt to the water which is soothing. Your doctor may also suggest other things he or she may want you to add to the water.

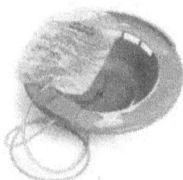

To prepare this, you can either use the plastic Sitz bath kit, (a special bowl specifically made for this which fits on your toilet seat so you can sit down easily on it), or your bath tub. Be sure to thoroughly scrub your plastic Sitz bath kit or bath tub before and after use. If using the bath tub, add sufficient warm water to sit on and then get in. To get the job done properly, you can try hanging your legs out of the tub. Usually, you are encouraged to sit for ten to fifteen minutes on the water. Pat the perineal area dry after you're done. Do not rub vigorously…remember the area is sore, and if you've had stitches, it could mess things up. This can be repeated up to three to four times daily as needed.

And now to the cord…

Do you wonder what to do with your baby's umbilical cord stump? How many times to clean it? What to clean it with? Methylated spirit, antiseptic lotion or water? Or perhaps you should just ignore it, hoping against hope that nature does its thing, and the stump falls off when it should, leaving your baby with a nice looking navel?

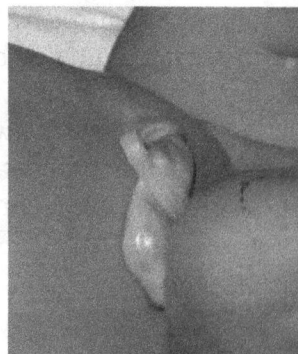

Well, a couple of years ago, the standard teaching was to wipe the stump with rubbing alcohol (methylated spirit) after every diaper change, but it was realized that this may have delayed the healing of the stump somewhat. The focus, really, is on keeping the stump clean and dry. Sterilize with clean water and then use absorbent paper or towel to pat dry. Rubbing alcohol may still be used, especially if baby was born premature or on your doctor's advice. Be sure to check with your doctor, what option to follow.

Be sure to clean this stump after every diaper change. Fold the front of the diaper to expose the stump to air and allow it dry naturally.

The stump usually goes through about three colour changes: yellowish green to brown and finally black. Allow the stump to dry up naturally and resist the temptation to pull off the stump even if it's hanging by less than a thread.

During the healing process, some pus or blood at the base may be observed. These are not signs to worry about. However, if the navel and surrounding area become inflamed (swollen, red and hot to touch), smelly and baby starts to run a fever, this may signify an infection, and you need to get your baby to see a doctor immediately.

Do cool mums breast feed?

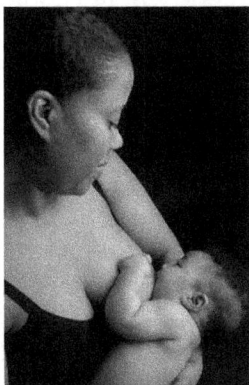

Whenever it's World Breast feeding week, it gets my mind racing down memory lane. A few years ago when I was pregnant for my first child, I made plans…loads of them. How great a mother I was going to be: I would make packed lunches, make her hair, teach her, school her, take her to work with me so I could exclusively breastfeed her, take her to school by myself (when it was that time), pick her up too, do her laundry by myself, etc. I wanted to be super mum. All those statistics of mothers who left their children was never going to be me and no child of mine was ever going to pass through that.

And so, I birthed this child. And, I set about doing all the things I had planned to do with a vengeance! I had no help…I insisted on doing everything myself. Never mind that by the end of the day I was frazzled, at my wits end and willing to bite people's ears off, if they so much as grazed past me, how much more touch a raw nerve! I also started looking for that hospital where I would work with my baby. I had just finished med school, house job and NYSC at that time, and so my head was brimming with all those ideas of bonding with my baby by breast-feeding and also ensuring I was giving her immune system a great boost for life…and all those wonderful reasons we were given for breast feeding.

In fact, as I was leaving med school, I was convinced that breast feeding was cool and oh so, fashionable! But the whole world conspired against me and all those noble ideals I had. I couldn't find any hospital that felt I was truly serious about working and discussing the concept of bringing my baby in and having a crèche where I could take off, now and again to breast feed and bond. In fact, none of those hospitals had crèches for their nursing-mother employees! Oh! Years later, I can imagine them bursting into gales of laughter anytime I left any of those interviews. 'Can you imagine? She wants to work…with a baby?!' 'Is she for real?!'

Thus started my reluctant stay-at-home period! It was to be for about two years. By this time, I had finally 'wised' up and figured that the society wanted mothers to breast feed their children, bond with them and reduce crime rates but no one was willing to make the sacrifice for that happen. And so, I made plans to put my daughter in school only to realise I was pregnant again. With my second daughter, breast feeding was perfunctory as I spent the period of pregnancy and immediately after birth plotting my return to the work place.

Having tried exclusive breast feeding and partial breast feeding, the difference was clear. Where my first daughter was a pillar of health during childhood, my second baby…though not sickly, always looked pale, picked up every virus flying around in the air and wasn't the easiest child to adapt to new diets.

Having experienced both extremes and becoming convinced about what made sense for me as a mother, I determined that with my next baby, I was going to work, (the housewife thing was not working for me. I was plain miserable! I doff my hat to all housewives! You're all amazing women and you rock!) and I was going to breast feed. And guess what? That was exactly what I did! I would breast feed at home and express regularly to freeze for the periods I was away at work. It wasn't easy but it was certainly worth it! So is it possible for a working mother? It is.

I smile when I hear working mothers say, "But I work, how can I do that?" You can, but it requires some sacrifice...actually lots of sacrifice. ● Breast milk, beyond being cheap, temperature regulated and readily available ☺ is formulated with everything your baby needs for each stage of his growth. It's chock full with vitamins, minerals, proteins, fats, oils and immunoglobulins which makes them resistant to illnesses. It is indeed a complete meal! It also helps the womb to return to normal size after childbirth.

Ladies, let's give our children the right start. It is still fashionable to breast feed. And even if not, who cares about what the fashion radar is saying on that, anyways!?! Or better still, let's start the fad!

Employers, please encourage this practice which is useful to society as a whole...crèches aren't such a bad idea when you think about the fact that you would now have dedicated female employees working for you.

PS: Ladies get some help at home. You know that 'super-mum' thing I was trying to do? It just exhausts you and you can't get it all done. Get a washing machine or someone to do the laundry. If you don't want a live-in help, get a daily. But whatever you do, get help! You'll be a lot happier. Trust me, I know!

Here's to a healthier, happier…and less stressed out you!

My food life… BC and AC

I remember those years before I had my first baby! I see some of those pictures and I gaze in awe. Those must have been the days when my mum would jokingly say I made skirts out of half a yard of fabric! I had my first baby and once she was six weeks old, I was back on the beat doing my exercises to get back to my BC (before child) status. My Yoruba aunt-in-law could not understand this and my utter lack of disregard for the plates of amala she attempted to serve up for my eating pleasure. I was determined to get back to my BC status and the earlier that happened, the better. This worked pretty well in this instance and before long, I was exactly how I wanted to be.

Then came along baby number two…and suddenly, it wasn't so easy to get back to my pre-pregnancy state. I managed it at the end of the day though…but it was with tightly gritted teeth, loads of sweat and oodles of perseverance. I realized at this time that my days of eating like a horse and burning it all off were gone. Oh, I used to be able to wolf down calories that even the fast food joints would shudder at, and not show a bit of spare flesh. What happened to that fantastic metabolic rate? It up and died on me because, it now appeared that even when I smelt food, I added weight! ☻ Honestly…I could almost swear!

Then came baby number three and my metabolism finally gave up. Every food I ate was duly converted to calories and stored in embarrassing areas of my body like my lower belly and my hips. I'm one of those lucky ones whose arms and wrists don't really 'swell' up whenever they add weight…but consider that I was unlucky in every other way as I added weight in every other place 😊 Again, I worked at it, even harder this time, and I was motivated by the fact that I'd been bought a couple of clothes to wear post pregnancy, and so they provided sufficient motivation to get with the crunches and sit-ups. And finally, the clothes fit!

In between, I tried some magic berry pills that were supposed to speed up your metabolism so fast it made your head spin! Mark you, I'm a doctor so I wasn't looking for anything that had any side effects that could affect my health. Nope, I wanted to do it naturally, but hey, if a pill helps, why not?! Yes? Well, I can tell you for a fact that my head spun, not from how fast my metabolism was converting fat to muscle but by how I could have ever considered there was an easier way…than sweating and grunting through it!

Did it get better afterwards? Nope, it became a constant battle to get the weight off and make it stay that way. I have this friend who wolves down everything in sight and yet, nothing happens. But not me! I finally made my peace with this new me…Ketch AC (After Children 👀) a couple of years ago and realized that this is my new reality…I add weight when I smell food 😁 So I can either stay down and whine about it or get up and do something about it.

And do something about it, I did. I committed to exercising at least five days every week or walking at least 7500 steps every day. I committed to reducing my portions and eating right. I made friends with beans, vegetables and fruits. Now, for some reason I never liked fruits. I could go for months (I think it would be absolutely embarrassing to say I could go for perhaps a year) without tasting (yes tasting…not even eating) a single fruit and then on some other occasions, I would get the craving for oranges and sit down with a knife in front of a basket of oranges and finish it off! I had to find a way of incorporating fruits into my diet. And that's when I really discovered smoothies. Now my life is not complete without my brew on a daily basis. I have even gone days on smoothies only...the weight just peeled off, and I assure you that even the most recalcitrant tummy would go flatter (depending on how much work has to be done, of course) on a diet of smoothies!

I'm not and never have been a huge fan of fad diets. I think they place a lot of restrictions on you that make them impracticable and thus easily abandoned. Therefore, for all of you who are wondering how to lose all that belly fat and asking if there's a magic pill, here's my answer. It is hard work...plain and simple.

First, focus on portion control. Start by reducing the size of your plate. If you eat with a bowl, go for a plate. If you eat with a flat plate with a circumference that could hold the globe 😊 go for a smaller one, etc. Then make sure that you focus on eating healthier foods. Half the plate should be filled with veggies, a quarter with protein and a quarter with carbs. Focus on complex carbs like brown rice, potatoes, yams, oats, etc. Your palm is actually a good measure of how much you should eat, and before you pelt me with rotten tomatoes for saying this, I've actually got very small palms, so I'm suffering through this too. 😊

Then, exercise. This could be in the gym or through your regular activities. If you are a stay-at-home mum, dancing while doing your house chores, may not be what you have in mind when you look at a full house of chores, but it could start you on your fitness journey. And if you have a house help, don't send her to do everything; get up and do some stuff yourself.

Taking a walk in the evening when everyone is back from work or school is also helpful. Going to the gym is a great way to start your day. In the office, move around some more...to the printer, to the bank, to the restaurant for lunch. Don't call for everything.

And then, try and reduce your stress level...I can almost hear your "yeah, right! How do I do that?" Well, stress is a normal part of life and, in fact, is needed to give you the regular push to get up and go every morning. Find out your sources of stress and figure out solutions to them. For those you can't find solutions for, let them go. No problem has ever been solved by stressing out over them. During stressful times, we are more likely to make wrong food choices. You may feel too lethargic to go anywhere and want to grab a quick food fix on your desk...where you've been sitting all day!

That's it...in as simple and plain a way as I could put it. These are the ABCs of losing weight...and we all keep working at it. I still have 1kg of my summer holiday weight left to lose before I continue my regimen from where I left off - did I really misbehave that much during the holidays? SMH

Join me and let's keep each other honest!

My tummy after my baby

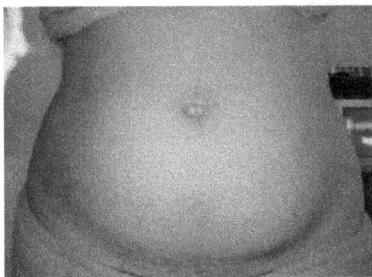

Hello pregnant mothers, or soon-to-be-pregnant mothers or husbands, brothers and friends of either pregnant or soon-to-be-pregnant mothers....yeah, yeah, I know! That was long winded, right?! I think old age is catching up with me. 😊

Okay, the most popular question I've received over time is how to lose the pregnancy-belly. Honestly, I've got no easy answers. It's diet and exercise...oh and breastfeeding. But breastfeeding is not very helpful if one is not exercising and watching their portions. Again, the dictum of feeding for two here doesn't count.

The diet to focus on is the very same one we talk about all the time: fruits, veggies and complex carbs with focus on healthier cooking methods (less frying and so on). Exercise should focus, initially on pelvic floor exercises especially if you're leaking urine when you cough or laugh. To locate your pelvic floor muscles, try holding your urine when you feel pressed. If you are successful, then you have located the muscles you need. Then empty your bladder and lie on the floor. Contract those same muscles and hold the contraction for about five seconds and then relax it for about five seconds. Gradually build this up to holding the contraction for ten seconds. Repeat this about three times a day. Once you no longer leak, you're ready for your exercises.

Have you noticed how it is usually easier to lose the baby weight after your first baby and harder afterwards? Focus on building up your stamina gradually especially if you were not very active in pregnancy or before. Please remember to always contact your doctor before starting any vigorous exercise program. As you get into the groove, get down with your aerobics, strength training and sit-ups et al.

This is where breast feeding comes in; if you're exercising and eating right, breastfeeding can help lose weight…as much as three hundred calories per day.

Does tying a wrapper tightly round your waist help flatten tummy? Honestly, I've heard people who swear by that technique. What I'll say is, if it works for you, why not? Just don't tie so tight as to stop blood flow.

How soon to start exercise after having a baby? Well, it depends on how active you were before and during pregnancy. If you were very active, you can start some light stretches as soon as you feel able. However, generally, we advise six to eight weeks after birth to allow for a post-natal check to have been done. Again, start small and allow your body to get into the groove.

And for all those who asked questions about breastfeeding, this should not be a problem, as once you position the baby correctly to the breast, milk is 'produced' for the baby through a let-down reflex. It is almost a misnomer to say one doesn't produce enough. It is not very common. So, nursing mothers should ensure that they drink copious amounts of water and put their babies to the breast. If breast feeding problems continue, see your doctor with your baby to ensure that the baby is latching on to the breast properly.

What's my baby saying when he's crying?

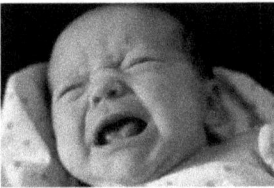
Are you a new mum trying to figure out what it all means? What's my baby saying when he whimpers, when he cries, when he screams (do you think, perhaps, someone pinched him?)…what does it all mean. It can be pretty overwhelming trying to make sense out of it all, I know.

Let's help you out: Here are some signals babies could be giving out when they cry.

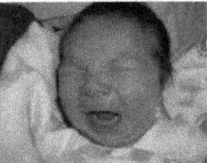
Hunger: If your baby isn't satisfied after a feed, he will cry at the end of it and before the next one. Babies also don't feel hungry at regular intervals and so there are days when he appears to need a feed more often and other days when he needs it infrequently. However, offer a feed if you're not sure what signal he is giving out.

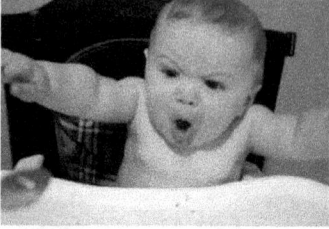

Needing to be held: We all worry about whether we will spoil our babies if we carry them whenever they cry. Well, if your baby needs a cuddle and that's why he is crying then you just need to carry him…and you won't spoil him! A front carrying baby sling may be a good idea. Otherwise, carrying or gently rocking your baby is also a good idea. Rocking is better than vigorously joggling him up and down because this may prevent him from drifting off to sleep. I made this mistake several times with my first baby and kept wondering why she never seemed to fall asleep!

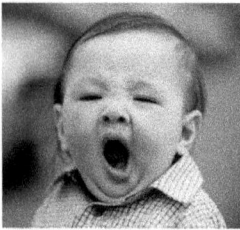

Tiredness: When a baby has had way too much excitement and stimulation, it can tire him out, making him irritable and unable to sleep. Make a habit of putting your baby down in a quiet, darkened room and leave him for a few minutes, even if he's crying, to see if he will settle and go off to sleep.

Too hot or too cold: You know those warm and woolly caps we wear on our children at all times, whether the weather is cold or hot? Bad idea!!! Babies can feel uncomfortably hot or cold, just as older children and adults do. If your baby is sweating or his tummy feels hot to the touch, remove some of his clothing. If he is in his cot, take off some of the bedding. Remove hats and extra clothing as soon as you come indoors or enter a warm car, bus or train. The room that a baby sleeps in should be neither too hot nor too cold. Please do not use a hot water bottle or electric blanket for your baby. Do not also place them in direct sunshine. These prevent overheating and significantly reduce the risk of cot-death as well making him more comfortable.

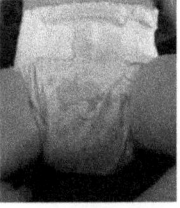

Wet or dirty nappies: Well, this bothers some children more than others! However, regardless of which category your child falls in, please change the nappy as soon as you realize it's wet or dirty. This helps to prevent nappy rash, which would almost certainly cause your baby discomfort.

Now you know what to do when your baby starts crying…let those maternal instincts kick in

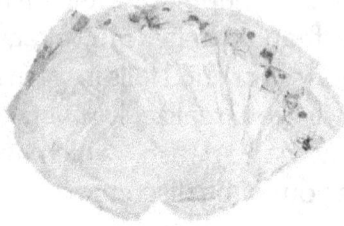

Diapering 101

My top tips for getting the diapering business right.

Ever started diapering your baby boy, only to be sprayed by a jet of urine? Yes, yes…I totally agree that it's a blessing as we say here in Africa, but you may well choose to do without this blessing if you're all dressed up and about to go out, right? When diapering a boy, it's a great idea to keep an extra cloth diaper close by to place over your baby's penis to catch those errant sprays. Having said that, still expect to get sprayed. It's just inevitable!!! (not very helpful, aye?!)

When diapering a girl, make sure you wipe from front to back to limit exposure to a urinary tract infection. And wash your baby's intimates with water more often than not. That's really all that is needed.

Leaking diapers suggest that diapers do not fit well around baby's legs. If you're experiencing a lot of leaks, it may be time to go up or back down a diaper size.

To prevent diaper rash:

- Change baby's diaper more often than you would normally do.
- Let baby's bottom air dry during a diaper change and if possible, leave

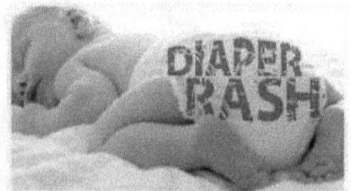

- the diaper off for a while.
- Use unscented, mild soap and a warm washcloth to clean baby during a diaper change. Perfumed and deodorant soaps can be harsh on baby's skin.
- If you use baby wipes, choose those that are free of perfume, alcohol, and chemicals.

Getting the right size of diaper for your baby is crucial as the diaper fits snugly around both the waist and legs, preventing leakage and also provides comfort as it is not tight enough to leave marks on baby's 'fragile' skin. Also be sure to go for un-perfumed brands to prevent irritations.

We are all aware that we should wash our hands thoroughly after changing a diaper, but you should wash up beforehand too. You should try to keep your hands clean anytime you'll be handling a baby, especially a new-born. Keep a hand sanitizer around the nappy changing area and in the diaper changing bag. Give your hands a quick cleaning before the change. Always remember to wipe baby from front to back and of course, wash-up when you are done!

You know the black, sticky, hard-to-remove poop your baby was producing soon after birth? It's called Meconium. After each diaper change, slather some petroleum jelly on baby's bottom to keep it nice and clean from meconium. The next time baby poops, the poop will slide right off!

If baby's bottom is irritated, try rinsing it off with a slightly warm spray of water from the sink or shower instead of using baby wipes that can actually irritate their little butts even further. Diaper rash ointment will work wonders and make baby feel better every time! If your baby is picky or fusses when you put it on, try putting some onto the diaper in a strategic location so it will connect with the irritated area once you close the diaper. 😄

Don't leave your baby alone and unattended when you are changing them on the changing table or any elevated surface even if you are using the safety straps. Please keep them safe. There are too many stories of babies left unattended who fell and sustained serious injuries. One second is all it takes. So, be careful!

Being a new mum can be daunting. But hey, you've got the most important ingredient needed to help your baby....love! We'll help out with the rest. 😄

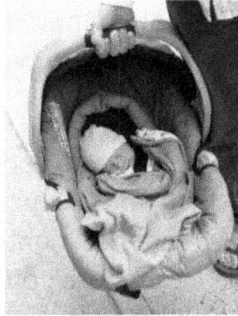

Planning an outing with baby?

Do you (new mum) often wonder what to pack in baby's diaper bag when you're going out? How much of everything you need or what you don't need at all?

Now let's help you out with the essentials you need to have in your baby's diaper bag...not suitcase.

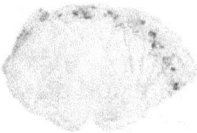

Diapers – be sure to pack enough diapers according to how often you change your baby...then add about two extra, just in case.

Diaper Rash Ointment – Whether your baby has a rash or not, always carry a small tube of Diaper Rash Ointment. Petroleum jelly is a good example. You just might open your baby's diaper and see the beginnings of a rash. The earlier you get to work treating it, the faster it will heal.

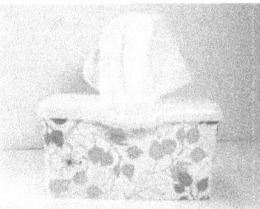

Wipes – A portable wipe bag is a life saver on many occasions...even when you're not carrying your baby. Oftentimes, you open your pack only to find that the wipes have dried out. Here's a tip for you: if you take them out and put them in a Ziploc bag, it seals in their moisture and freshness, and is, of course, easier to pack in the diaper bag. Genius, right?

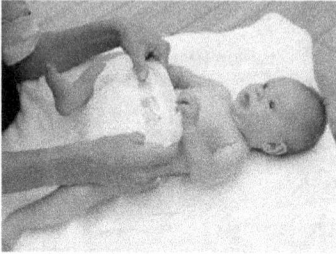

Changing Pad – Now you need a surface to put your baby down to change him/her right? There are two options: either use your own changing pad or buy disposable changing pads. Carrying around the changing pad you use at home is cumbersome, and you would be putting it down in places that may be breeding with germs. Afterwards, these germs are transferred to your diaper bag as you put your changing pad back into the bag. The disposable ones are easier to pack, and you throw them away after use. Pack at least as many disposable changing pads as you pack diapers. You can buy disposable changing pads in big supermarkets.

Make sure you wash your hands afterwards to ensure that you do not infect yourself, your baby or indeed your family with germs.

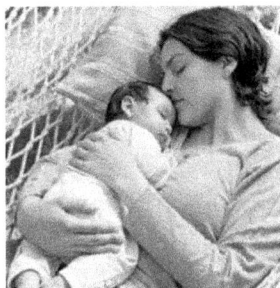

Rest for new mums...joke, right?

For those new mummies with children, this may be more wishful thinking as our bundles of joy have minds of their own. 😊 We just wish sometimes that we could explain nicely to them that we....well, just need to sleep now; regardless of how much they want to chat or cry especially in the middle of the night! Well, we've some helpful tips that ensure a good night's rest for mum and new baby.

During night-time feedings, keep lights low. Night lights stop you and baby from coming fully awake and so you can go back to sleep after the feed...effortlessly.

Commit to sleep and make it a priority in your life. The advice frequently given to new mothers to get some sleep when the baby is asleep, may sound clichéd, just like 'an old wives' tale, but is useful. Give yourself permission to let some things go and don't feel the pressure to catch up on all your emails, text messages, house chores when he's asleep.

Good sleep starts before you're actually trying to fall sleep. Ensure you start winding down your day early enough so you can get to sleep early at night. Ensure you're not getting too wound up during the day and messing with your ability to sleep at night.

As a new mother, you've got so many things pulling at you: night time feeds, your other children, (if you've got them), their homework, your husband, etc. So ensure that your sleep equipment – pillows, mattress pad/topper and mattress – provide the right support and comfort. Get a good pillow and comfortable mattress…it's a worthwhile expense.

Be open to alternative remedies. Create a personal spa at home: use aromatic oils at bath time and in your room. Lavender has been found to be very helpful by some.

Remember that brilliant ideas grow in rested minds. So, get rested and keep loving your precious bundle of joy.

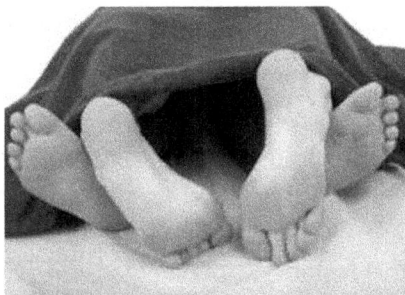

When to resume sexual relations after a baby?

The honest answer is, as soon as you and your spouse feel up to it. Usually, six weeks is advocated at which time the woman would have had a post-natal check. However, there is really no scientific basis for this and the time a woman feels like intimacy could differ from woman to woman.

Some women feel ready earlier and some much later. Bear in mind that there are new issues contending for attention here…namely the new baby who requires a lot of attention, the overwhelming emotion of being in charge of a new life especially for new mothers, the sheer exhaustion after looking after the baby's needs and sleep deprivation, the pain of vaginal suturing(if the woman had a tear), the dryness of the vagina at this time, etc. We could go on and on! With all these, it may be difficult to feel really sexy…trust me, I know.

So, what's the way forward? New mums, get as much help as you can so that you don't feel exhausted every night. Also, rest whenever the baby is taking a nap. Perhaps, periods for intimacy can also be re-scheduled to other times…maybe mornings while the baby is still sleeping. Then again, you don't have to wait for full sexual intercourse to be intimate. You can start off with cuddling and then move on to more adventurous things. Lubrication may also be a great idea to help with vaginal dryness.

To help restore muscular tone to the vagina, pelvic floor exercise (Kegel exercises) should be started as soon as possible. The exercise mimics the movements we make when we want to stop the flow of urine. Try to hold this for about ten seconds and then doing about four or five repetitions per set. Try about three sets per day and increase this as you feel ready.

Remember to use birth control even if you're breastfeeding exclusively. You don't want to get pregnant while nursing a baby, right? 😊

Fact or Fiction

This book will not be complete without writing about those amazing pieces of advice that people have repeated and passed along through various eras that they have practically taken the place of the truth! I will address some of them and let you know our verdict...fact or fiction.

Advice
You must always have a safety pin on your person otherwise evil people may steal the baby from your tummy.

Verdict: Fiction
I'm not sure how else to qualify this, except by saying it is beyond weird!

Advice
Do not let people cross your leg when you're sitting down. If they do, your baby will look like them.

Verdict: Fiction
Seriously guys! This has no basis in reality and even in mythology. If you don't like people crossing over your legs, that's fine...but don't get it twisted. It has nothing to do with how the baby looks.

Advice
Do not spend too much time or shout at people you don't like or your baby will look like them.

Verdict: Fiction
Anything that gets you to stop screaming is a great idea. But let's do it for the right reasons. Your baby's looks are determined by genes and not your likes or dislikes.

Advice

If you scream during labour for your first child, you will scream throughout all your other labours.

Verdict: Fiction

Honestly, if you'd like to give your lungs a work-out during labour, be my guest. Go for it. I really don't see any problem in it...certainly no documented medical one. In my case, to make up for the two times I tried to keep it all in, as I'd mentioned, I screamed the whole neighbourhood down when I was having my last baby! But then again, you really don't need to scream. You can give birth to your baby in a centre where you can receive epidural anaesthesia so that the whole process is easy-peasy, lemon-squeezy.

In Africa, we like to think that if we don't have our babies the long, painful way, it makes us less of women. But that is not true. The woman who had her baby with anaesthesia and the woman who didn't both have babies to show for their efforts and I assure you that in both cases, the maternal instincts are not affected.

Advice

'If the doctors tell you that the best option for you is to have your baby through a Caesarean section, reject it. All the women in our families have had their babies 'normally' and you can't be an exception to that rule.'

Verdict: Fiction

Every woman's story is different and so is their medical history. Your mum's history is not necessarily yours and so, judging what will happen to you at labour and delivery by what happened to your family before you, may be putting you in danger. In some instances, there may not even be a problem with a woman's ability to deliver the baby, but because the labour is prolonged with the baby in distress, the doctor takes a decision to section the lady. Going against this advice (which is an option open to the woman as the doctor will not force his medical opinions on her) may endanger both mother and baby. So, please be guided.

Advice
If you eat a lot of snails, your baby will spit a lot when born!

Verdict: Fiction
The fact that the snail is slimy has nothing to do with whether baby drools or not. Remember also that if your baby starts drooling when he's teething, it has nothing to do the with the snails you ate when pregnant but everything to do with the process he's going through...bringing forth teeth!

Advice
A breastfeeding mother cannot get pregnant.

Verdict: Fiction
This actually was used as a birth control method called the Lactational Amenorrhea Method (LAM), because the hormones involved in lactation, provide some protection against pregnancy-related hormones. However, we have seen time and again, women get pregnant while breasfeeding to know that this is not a reliable method of birth control!

Advice
A pregnant mother must not breastfeed.

Verdict: Fiction
Much as it would have been a great idea to be completely done with one baby before starting on another one, the breastfeeding does not affect the baby in the womb. So, do not

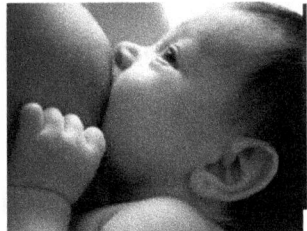

deprive your new-born baby of his or her 6 months of exclusive breast-feeding.

Advice
Pregnant women should not sleep on their backs as this may damage your baby's eyes.

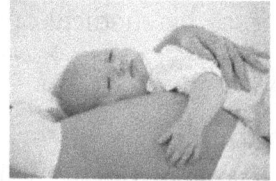

Verdict: Fact and Fiction
In the first trimester, if you're used to sleeping on your back, you can continue. However, as you get into your second trimester, it is a fact that pregnant women should not sleep on their backs especially close to term. However, the reason is not because of damage to baby's eyes. It's because the woman may feel dizzy as the growing uterus puts pressure on the vein that returns blood from the body making the woman feel dizzy on getting up and the baby may also not get enough nutrients from the placenta in that position.

Advice
If a pregnant woman drinks cold water, her baby may get pneumonia.

Verdict: Fiction
Seriously?! It's fictional enough the fact that we think that in real life, cold water drinking exposes us to pneumonia, but an unborn child....seriously?! This is as fictional as it gets. No basis in truth.

Advice
No sex during pregnancy.

Verdict: Fiction
This is one advice that I'm sure a lot of people are pleased to know is fictional. Of course, the couple may have to get inventive with comfortable positions based on the woman's growing

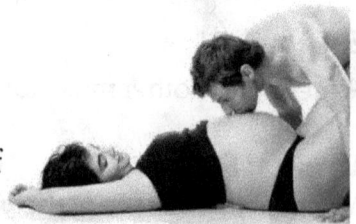

tummy. However, depending on the woman's medical history, it may be a good idea also to check with the woman's doctor that there are no issues that can pose a problem to this.

Advice
If you're carrying low, it's a boy and if you're carrying high, it's a girl.

Verdict: Fiction
In the early days of pregnancy, pregnancies are carried high and later as delivery time approaches, the baby's head engages in the pelvis in preparation for birth. So, if we were to believe this, it means everyone carries a girl early in pregnancy...who now becomes a boy before birth? Kind of confusing, right? And then, what is the story for the people who eventually end up having girls having been told they had low carrying bellies?

This has no basis in fact!

Advice
If you have a lot of morning sickness, then it's a girl.

Verdict: Fiction
There's absolutely no basis in truth here. You can be sick every single day of your pregnancy whether you're having a boy or girl.

Advice
I am pregnant and my first scan showed that I have fibroid. I want to know if I should stop taking Folic Acid as I heard that it may make the fibroid become bigger.

Verdict: Fiction
Fibroids do not feed on folic acid...they feed on hormones that is the

reason why they may become bigger in pregnancy and tend to shrink during menopause. Please ensure that you take your folic acid so as to ensure your baby has no neural tube (spinal cord) defects and be sure that your pregnancy is being supervised by an obstetrician.

Advice
There are calculations and positions that can make you have a baby boy or girl.

Verdict: Fiction
There are calculations using the rhythm method that try to pinpoint the exact day of ovulation and encourage sexual intercourse on that day for a male child. This is theoretical at best and is not a fool-proof way of having a male or female child.

The other gist about positions is even more hilarious!

Advice
Don't eat snails or your labour will be too rapid.

Verdict: Fiction
Again, this focuses on the sliminess of the snail to make this claim. Rapid or precipitate labour has nothing to do with eating snails or not. Nobody really knows why this happens beyond linking some risk factors like unusually small babies, roomy pelvic outlets (outlet for passage of the baby), etc.

Advice
Put a stone at the end of your wrapper and knot it when going out to prevent miscarriage.

Verdict: Fiction
Really!!! This is truly without any basis in science and pushes fiction too far.

Advice
Don't eat plantain when pregnant or the baby's anterior fontanelle (the depression in the front of the head) will be very deep.

Verdict: Fiction
Baby's anterior fontanelle would be deep or depressed if the baby is dehydrated and not because the mother loves dodo!

Advice
The first breast milk, colostrum, should be discarded as it is dirty and causes rashes in children

Verdict: Fiction
Colostrum is the first milk produced by the mother and is loaded with antibodies and nutrients needed by the baby. Babies should not be deprived of this milk.

Advice
Women should not take the prenatal vitamins given at the hospitals because it makes babies grow unnecessarily big.

Verdict: Fiction
The iron tablets are important to prevent anaemia (blood shortage) in pregnant women and the folic acid ensures that baby's spine develops well with no defects. In fact, it is advised that women who wish to get pregnant should start taking folic acid about three months before they conceive.

Advice

Pregnant women should not drink directly from the bottle so that baby will not have hiccups

Verdict: Fiction

Well, it certainly is a great idea to be lady-like and drink from a cup, right But this has nothing to do with baby having a hiccup.

Advice

Pregnant women should eat native clay called nzu in Ibo. This helps wash unborn baby's body so that when born the baby is very clean. It also stimulates an appetite in these pregnant women.

Verdict: Fiction

Eating loads of clay will only end up giving you constipation, can potentially harm your baby and where there is a craving for it, it may even be suggestive of iron deficiency anaemia.

Advice

Presence of a black line below the navel can tell you if the baby is a boy or girl.

Verdict: Fiction

Presence or absence of a black line says nothing about the sex of the baby. If you wish to know this, an ultrasound scan will do the magic.

Advice

Pregnant women who deliver in hospitals are not brave.

Verdict: Fiction

This has led to a situation where women who ought to seek medical care in the hospital stay home to prove they are brave. Please be sure to register for your antenatal classes, attend regularly and follow your doctor's advice to the letter.

Advice
Having sexual intercourse on specific days of the menstrual cycle guarantees having a boy or a girl

Verdict: Fiction
Well, this used to be popularly propagated...tongue twister, right?! ; 😉 But here's the truth, the whole truth and nothing but the truth...this matter is completely in God's hands. Some people who go for some forms of assisted reproduction may be offered the choice of picking their baby's sexes, but even this is not routinely done.

So cherish your gifts from God, boy or girl...and love them to bits 😊

Final Advice
Don't worry about the pregnancy pain. As soon as you have your baby, all the pain will magically melt away.

Verdict: Fact
This is one advice I am so happy to tell you is all fact and no fiction. once the baby is born, the physical pain pales in significance when compared to the emotional joy and happiness of having your baby...most times. Be sure to hold on to and treasure all your memories with your baby(ies) because sooner than you think they are all grown up and leaving home.

There are many more myths making the rounds. Do you know anyone we haven't used here? Drop me a line and it could be included in the next edition of this book 😊

Let's rid the world of silly myths that endanger the lives of our women. Join me?

PARENTING

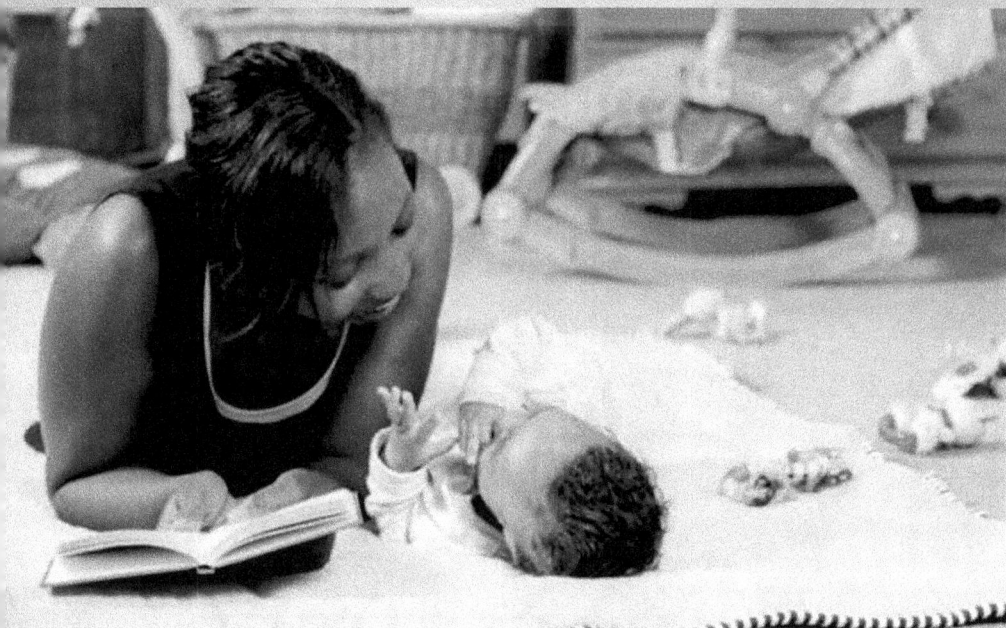

FOR THE

UNINITIATED!

PARENTING

for the

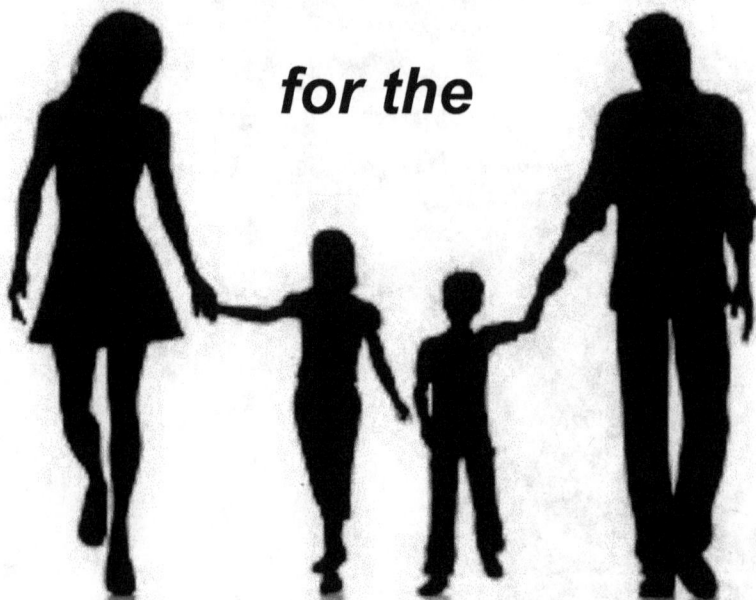

UNINITIATED!

Table of Contents

Introduction

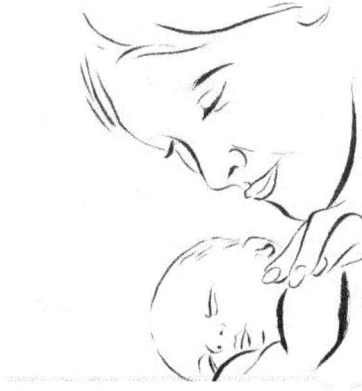

Parenting! Not the easiest of jobs, aye?

And we are constantly learning! I tell my first daughter that she will always be my learning curve because I experienced motherhood for the first time through her, and I pass through every stage of her life, learning what it feels like for the first time.

I remember her first day in nursery school. I was so excited. My daughter was going to a proper school for the first time. This clearly set me apart from all the other mothers that still had their children in reception or creches. And then she graduated…yes, graduated - from nursery school, no less! 😊

The day she started attending Primary School, I thought my heart was going to burst with pride. I kept looking around to see if everyone had observed that my level had changed. I now had a child in Primary school.

Immediately after dropping the Nursery school crew, I moved on to the big school. My goodness, I had arrived! 😊

I remember her first party at school! I went to town, bought her the prettiest dress I could find and decked her out in it with bows and ribbons et al. She looked like a bejewelled princess.

Imagine my shock when we got to school, and I saw other children very casually dressed in jeans and tees! It was now a case of 'were they under-dressed?' or 'were we over-dressed?'
Well, the activities of the day were helpful in clearing this up. Class party days were fun periods dedicated to bouncy castles and all manner of entertainment that involved jumping up and down. Definitely, not the sort of activities I had in mind when I was convinced that she had to be a bejewelled princess. 😊

And so, this was one of my first lessons but by no means the last I learnt with my first child. The other mummies already had other children (who they had probably gotten their schooling from) or perhaps friends who advised them better. 😊

I'm sure you're wondering what I did when it was time for Secondary School…I could not wait to tell everyone. This was not one of those instances where you wished and hoped that people noticed a change of status. Oh no! I told everyone who cared to listen and people who were also minding their business.I found a way of interjecting the gist into every conversation, and I'm sure people found me an absolute bore! 😊

The Lord help you all when my kids get into the university. That will certainly inspire another book! 😊

And, the learning continues. Of course, I have picked up many other lessons with my first daughter and continue to acquire knowledge. Every time we started something for the first time, I learnt how to do it and how not to. And so with my other two children, I looked like a pro to all the other mothers. They oftentimes asked me how I knew all about this stuff and I laughed so hard when they were not looking…if only they knew! 😊

Well, this is a collection of my ramblings about the continually evolving state of parenthood. I'll share with you my journey as it has been so far…and as usual, my take on some of the questions that were sent to my social media pages. But hey, perhaps, you all get to learn from my goofs, so you don't have to make as many mistakes as I did. 😊

I start off with a message that is not strictly about parenting. It is really about the decision we make before we become parents. I hope you get the points embedded therein and help make our children's lives much easier.

I hope you enjoy reading it. Please drop me an email.

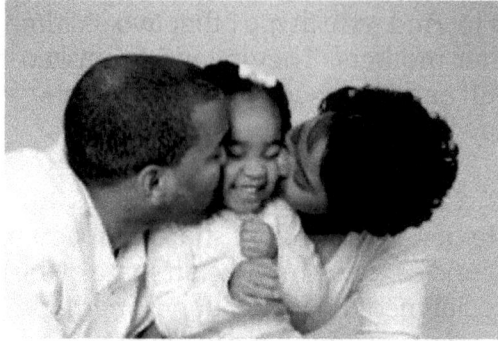

Long Before The Parenting....

Love is blind…is it?

Did you enjoy reading Mills and Boon and all the tales about falling in love in the good old days? The dashing tall, dark and handsome men who were to charge into our lives with panache and sweep us off our feet. 😜 Some of us got the 'Prince Charming' (on white horses, to boot) and some of us did not. But, hey hold it…this book is not about that!

It is about the things that love supposedly makes us do! I checked up an online dictionary, and it defines love as an intense feeling of deep affection. Hmm! Then I went a step further and checked up the meaning of blindness and this online source tells me that this is a state of being sightless and unable to see. So, if love is blind, it prevents anyone with this feeling of deep affection from seeing…literally and figuratively! Hmm, thoughts to ponder. I'll leave this discourse here for a bit and move on to another issue.

Parenthood is a huge job. It involves a human being literally sacrificing all for another person. You want to protect your children from pain, hurts and losses, even when you know it is impossible. When they are ill, you want to take over the illness and leave them well. So imagine if you were the parent of a sickle-cell patient, who has to deal with health crisis, pain and is really sickly most of the time.

You are constantly praying to God to please reduce the pain, and indeed you are in the hospital more often than not with this child.

How did this happen, you wonder? Well, it was when two sickle-trait carriers (people with AS) decided to get married. This automatically meant that they had a 25% chance that any child they had would have Sickle Cell Disease (genotype SS). This is a mathematical probability, and it could very well be that none of this couple's children would be SS, or it could very well be that all or half of them could be SS! So imagine starting out on a journey of parenthood knowing that your heart is going to break repeatedly as you deal with your child's continual visits in and out of the hospital.

Now where is the link up with the old wives tale of love being blind? It was World Sickle Cell day, recently, and it got me wondering about this thing called love. Well, I think that love should not be blind…not in these times where there are all sorts of sources for generating power. ☻

More seriously, love really has no choice than to be pragmatic these days, therefore, before marriage, a couple should be sure to carry out tests. I am not talking about those carried out by churches to confirm pregnancy, but a serious desire by couples to seek answers as they make the decision to undertake a voyage together. This should ideally be done or known by both parties early enough in a relationship before emotional investments are made on either side. If two people are carriers of the sickle cell trait, it is only sensible not to marry.

Before you all lynch me, I know it is not as easy as it sounds. But marrying because you are emotionally invested even though you know the status is really exchanging one type of heartbreak for another…because your heart will surely break when you are forced to watch your child go through the pains of the many crises he or she will have to deal with or worse still, to have them die in your hands.

If I were to choose, I most definitely know what the choice would be for me. It may not be an easy choice, but we have got to break the trend of these increasing numbers of sicklers in our communities. If ignorance is the problem, let's spread the knowledge; if love being blind is the problem, ladies and gentlemen, please bring a flashlight along and show the light!

Here is to a healthier generation and a healthier you!

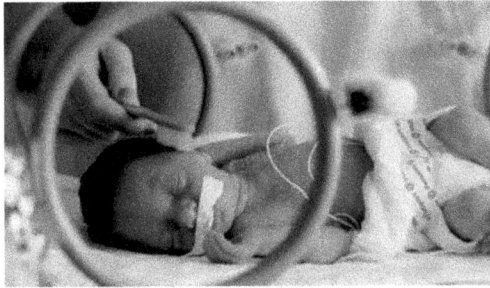

Prematurity Awareness

November of every year is prematurity awareness month.

What is prematurity? A premature baby comes into the world before thirty-seven completed weeks of pregnancy. Babies born prematurely have to be in intensive care (Special Care Baby Unit) so as to give them a fighting chance. They are prone to having problems like apnoea (where the baby sometimes stops breathing), anaemia (shortage of a sufficient number of red blood cells to take oxygen round the body), respiratory problems and low-blood pressure, etc.

Who is at risk of having a premature baby? Sometimes we don't really know the cause, but it has been observed in mothers younger than nineteen years of age and older than forty years.

Some cases can be brought on by chronic diseases which the mother already had before pregnancy like Hypertension and Diabetes or could be due to Urinary Tract Infections, abnormal positions of the placenta during gestation or multiple pregnancies involving carrying more than one baby in the womb e.g. twins. Smoking, drinking alcohol, drug abuse and failure of the mother to feed well during pregnancy are other factors that can lead to prematurity.

So, once you get pregnant start your ante-natal classes as soon as possible and let your doctor know if you have any of the mentioned risk factors. In the developing countries like Nigeria, our survival rates for prematurity (depending on the number of completed weeks of pregnancy) are not as good as in advanced countries.

Let's give our babies a fighting chance.

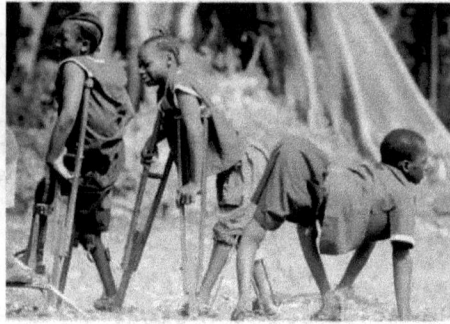

Make Polio a failure!

A couple of years ago, I was notified of a case that involved one of the hospitals on our private Health Insurance Scheme and the child of one of our enrollees. This child had a fever that had been running for a couple of days; the parents were not comfortable anymore and decided to go to the hospital. Predictably, the hospital decided to place this child on antibiotics irrespective of the fact that nothing pointed to the fact that this was anything more than a viral infection.

This child could have taken the drugs orally or very well have swallowed this unnecessary antibiotic by mouth, but for some reason - whether by request from the child's parents who wanted something they perceived to be more potent or as a show of 'we know what we are doing here' by the hospital staff - a decision was made to administer this drug through intramuscular injection (in English, injection into the muscle...in this case, the buttocks specifically).

To cut a long story short, a short while later we got involved as we received a letter from the company of the child's parent stating that the hospital was incompetent and administered an injection that caused the child to lose function of her lower limbs. We stepped in and eventually, the gist of the story was that this child was incubating the wild polio virus and the intramuscular injection this child had received converted this to paralytic polio! In a short space of time, this child now found it difficult to walk. Just like that!!!

Okay, why am I telling this story? Well, every 24th of October is World Polio Day and as the event to mark the day were rolled out this time, I thought about this case I had just told you about, and I wondered about that child and how much use of her limbs she has now. And then I wondered about other parents who coerce their health care providers to give 'stronger' medicines in the form of injections so that their children would get better, quicker? How many healthcare providers fall for this 'persuasion' or even sometimes, downright 'instructions' from their patients or patients' parents? How many even have an idea how Polio is transmitted and how they can effectively guard against this? If you don't have the right knowledge, you will fall for anything.

A good example of this is a story I heard a couple of years ago about a quack practitioner somewhere in the country who made money off hardworking traders by claiming that he could help them wash out the impurities in their blood.

For the people who fell for this scam, he would admit them into his 'hospital' and then set up an infusion with diuretics in it. In simple terms, diuretics are drugs that make you urinate a lot. The guy also proceeded to attach a urinary catheter (a tube that collects urine from a person's bladder into a urine bag) to the tubes so that the patients could see the quantity of urine their bodies were making. The impurities were meant to be in the vast amounts of urine being poured out!

I am just shaking my head at the amazing gullibility and ignorance that makes us fall for anything and makes unscrupulous people take advantage of us. By the way, this guy was picked up by the police some time back.

But, I digress…back to the Polio discourse.

How is the polio virus spread? It is spread through faeco-oral contact. I will describe this.

A child with the wild polio virus defecates and sheds the virus in his or her 'poo'. These faeces can contaminate water sources or can get into food as a result, of inappropriate or lack of hand washing and basic hygiene. Once one case is diagnosed, it is thought to be an epidemic already as one can be a carrier of the virus for a long time before symptoms actually show. The initial symptoms include fever, tiredness, headache and limb or neck stiffness.

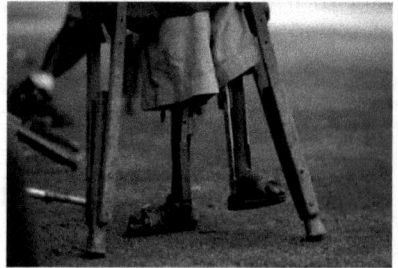

Not everyone infected with the virus actually develops paralytic disease. There are some pre-disposing factors to the development of paralytic disease, and they include intramuscular injections (like the baby in the story above), injuries, strenuous exercise, pregnancy, immune deficiency and removal of tonsils.

Does this mean we should trash our exercise routine (you wish☺) or not get pregnant (let's watch you convince your spouse☺)? The point being made is that these groups of people are prone to this and should ensure that they practice proper hygiene and sanitation to prevent it, given its mode of transmission.

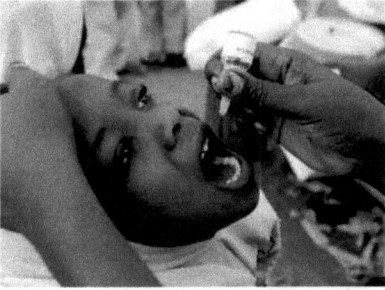

All children below the age of five years should be immunized and booster doses given whenever the Government sends out her officials to do so. It's not cool to send them away as if they are some troublesome 'pests' disturbing your peace. Their jobs save lives. If enough children are immunized, the cycle of infection can be broken, and our children will live healthier, longer and better lives. Remember, there's no cure for polio…only treatment to deal with the symptoms.

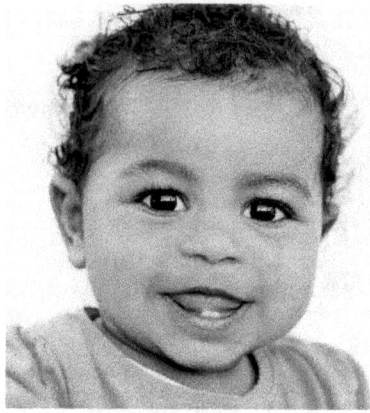

Teething In Babies

Have you ever heard that when children start teething, they start stooling? I am sure we have all heard that at one time or the other, but guess what? There's no research that has shown any link between the process of erupting a tooth and diarrhoea. If anything, we have found out that this is the same period when children start picking up things and, of course, the natural 'tourist' destination for anything they pickup is their mouths! 😃 What happens? When they pickup dirty stuff and suck on it, it would ultimately lead to diarrhoea.

So, more than ever, that's the time to be watchful and ensure that the children are not stuffing their mouths with rubbish as well as ensure their toys are cleaned.

Having said that, how can I help my baby through the teething phase, especially with the itch and discomfort they feel around the 'erupting tooth' area? Even the drooling? Well, here are a few things you could do:

- Rub over the teething area with your finger (thoroughly scrubbed and clean, of course ☺) or use a finger covered with clean gauze or even the baby's wash cloth. If this is cool to touch, it is even better. Massage the teething area with this as it helps to soothe the discomfort.

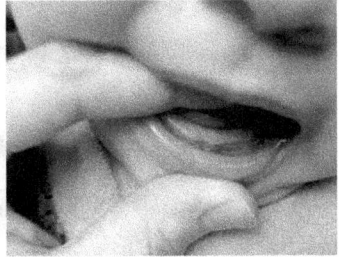

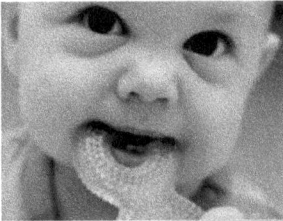

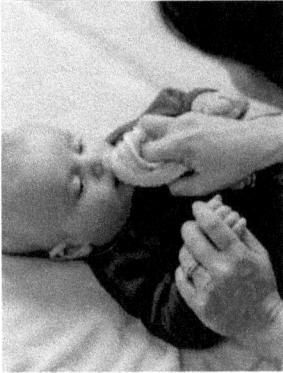

- Teething rings are great ideas too, and you could also refrigerate these to provide more comfort but please do not freeze them.

- Clean off the drooling saliva as this could cause irritation around the baby's mouth, worsening his crankiness.

- Over the counter analgesics could also be helpful provided it's given in the appropriate dose for the baby's age. Please avoid Aspirin as it causes a disease called Reye's syndrome.

- Although several studies have been conducted on the efficacy of gripe water it has not really been found to be particularly useful in teething but it is liberally used by parents and doctors alike. Older formulas contained alcohol which was thought to be perhaps, responsible for the soothing effect it had; however, other components like the herbs may not go down well with all children.

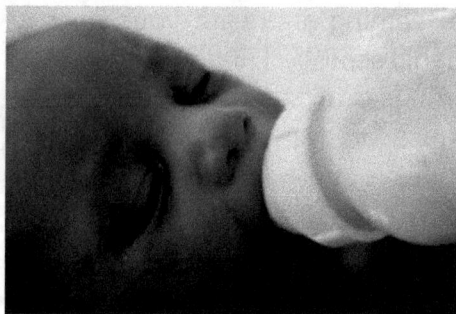

Baby Bottle Tooth Decay

The baby bottle tooth decay is a condition that occurs when babies' teeth are exposed to prolonged contact with sugary liquids or substances. In children, this would occur when they are allowed to go to sleep while feeding at the breast, on a bottle or giving them pacifiers that have been coated with honey or other sugary substances.

During sleep, saliva production decreases thus, these sugary substances which lead to the production of acids stay on the teeth for prolonged periods leading to erosion of the enamel and subsequent tooth decay.

To keep this condition at bay;

- Mothers are advised to practice exclusive breastfeeding but if bottles have to be used for any reason during that period, this should be carefully monitored. Please ensure the baby never falls asleep while nursing on the breast or bottle containing milk (be it expressed breast milk or formula), fruit juice (fresh or packaged) or any other sweetened fluids. This ensures that the baby's teeth is not in contact with

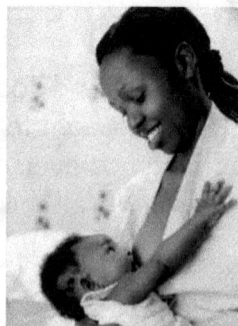

- sugary fluids for prolonged periods of time and prevents tooth decay.

- Clean baby's mouth and gums at least once a day, gently massaging the gingival tissues and gum. It can be done using a piece of moistened cotton gauze wrapped around a finger. This helps to clean baby's mouth, establish the development of healthy teeth and also aid teething.

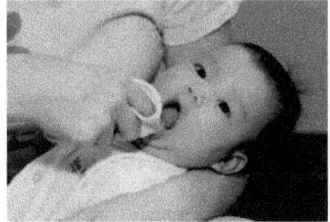

- As soon as the first tooth erupts, plaque removal should commence. Make sure your babies' teeth are brushed at least twice a day. Before a child learns to spit out, please use a non-fluoride containing toothpaste. We don't want the child swallowing fluoride and coming down with some ailments. However, as soon as the child can spit saliva on their own, please introduce fluorinated toothpaste.

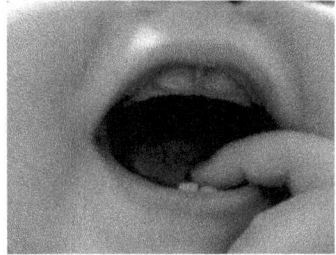

- Wean the baby from the bottle as soon as possible and use a cup for liquids. During the weaning period, dilute the bottle feeds as much as possible to the point where only water is taken with the bottle.

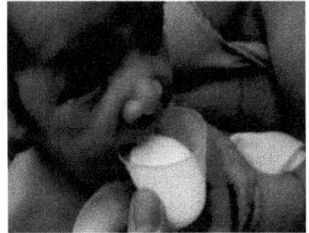

- If your baby uses a pacifier, please use for only short periods of time and be sure not to coat with honey or any other sugary substance to ensure that his teeth are not in prolonged contact with substances that will lead to tooth decay.

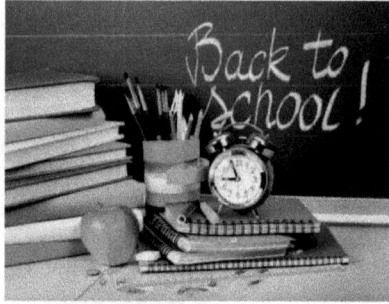

Back-to-School Tool Kit

Whenever it's time to go back to school, shops that specialize in school uniforms and stationery do brisk business. Daddies and mummies dig deep to pay the outrageously exorbitant fees that pass for school fees these days (please forgive me if you own a school. I'm actually 'seriously' considering starting one myself 😊).

Anyways, as they say, 'better soup, na money kill am!' For the benefit of my 'aje-butter' friends, that means that (the) quality (of soup) is determined by the funds committed (or in the soup's case, the funds that went into procuring the ingredients). Okay…certainly long winded, but I guess the meaning came across; yes? Stay with me (and bear with me 😊); I'm aging so I tend to use ten words where two could have worked! 😊

The weather appears to change at will. I am so muddled up with the seasons these days. When I was growing up, dry and rainy season were so clearly defined that you always knew what to expect at any time…not anymore. Kudos to global warming and climate change! With the changing of the weather, usually come 'the sniffles.'

Do you have a child who appears to catch anything that just moves around in the air? They go to school and will catch a cold provided another child has it? They will get measles, just by looking at a child that has one...even from a safe distance (okay...that's an exaggeration that was meant to make you smile 😊). I had one of those; my daughter would pick up any virus that was making the rounds! My constant prayer every day was, 'Lord don't let this child die.'

And so I decided to take things personal. When she was in a creche, I led a campaign to ensure that children who had the sniffles were kept home and not dumped on unsuspecting caregivers in the school. It would amaze you how many mothers do this. I am not passing judgment here because a lot of parents have to work and so staying home to look after a sick child may not be an excuse that is readily understood by bosses. But, the child risks having a medical emergency in school that cannot be handled by caregivers and, of course, poses a threat to other children who were previously uninfected. If the roles were reversed, you certainly don't want your child going to school and picking up other people's germs.

I worked with the creche to ensure that all hand held toys were disinfected every morning and after use by the children as their use of the hand held toys (at the creche stage) simply involved dipping the toy into their mouths and sucking for dear life! Flu and other droplet infections are spread by contact with droplets from someone else who has an infection.

At the primary level, anytime I am invited to give talks, I focus on droplet infections and how they are spread. I teach the children how to wash their hands, for at least twenty seconds, preferably using running water and hot air for drying.

The steps to effective hand washing in the 'perfect' situation are:

- Wet hands with clean running water and apply soap.

- Rub your hands together to make a lather and then scrub between fingers, under the nails and the back of your hands.

- Continue to scrub for at least twenty seconds.

- Rinse your hands under running water.

- Dry off with a clean towel or hot air dryer.

Okay, not every convenience has a hot air dryer or even running water; if you've got one of those toilets, just ensure that you pour the clean water on to sudsy hands and scrub for twenty seconds…that's the time it takes to sing Happy Birthday twice or really the time it takes to scrub your hands, front, back and in between fingers and nails!
Remember to teach your children that germs hide in every single nook and cranny. They are on the toilet handles, the tap knob, the tissue dispenser, etc. Thus, after using the toilet, wash your hands last after you have cleaned yourself up and flushed.

Okay, I heard that snigger…'yeah right!… like anyone has to be taught that!'

Well, actually, quite a number of people have to be taught as we have realized that quite a number of children are not trained early enough and would have come down with some diseases before they know it.

Buy them hand sanitizers. Alcohol based sanitizers reduce the number of germs on hands. The children can use these even after washing their hands and leaving the toilet, in cases where there was insufficient water. In addition, this is a handy tool for all those times they come in contact with 'eewyeeckies' and don't have the luxury of washing their hands when they have been shaken by someone they just observed sneezing into their hands, etc. The small handy packs of sanitizers fit well into most pencil cases. [The sanitizer should be applied to the palm of one hand, both hands rubbed together and product rubbed over the surface of hands and fingers until the hands are dry]. Sanitizers that contain at least 60% alcohol are most effective, especially when water and soap are not readily available.

Teach them to sneeze into the crooks of their arms and not into their palms. With this, we will be building the next generation of people who do not go around sneezing (rendering thousands of germs homeless) in people's faces (finding alternative homes for these germs) or into their hands and then subsequently shaking other people's hands (ensuring that these germs hit their mark).

Back-tracking to toilet training again, teach the children especially the girls, to clean from the front backwards. Many an infection has been caused by faecal matter deposited in places where they have no business being! Girls should also be taught to clean up after urinating as early as possible. This can also aid to prevent infections that thrive in warm and moist places like Candida.

So, beyond the books, stationery and inevitable school fees, let us ensure that our children have the right health and wellness toolkit to survive a new term and come home with those amazing grades we all look forward to!

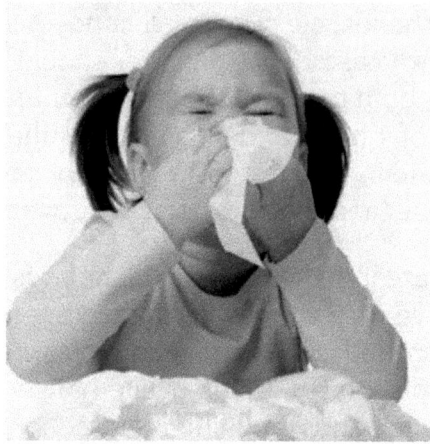

The Sniffles Are Here!

My daughter came back one day complaining of sore throat. I figured she was about to come down with a cold, and I kept asking her if she had 'the sniffles'. At that time, she didn't have that but she could not understand, for the life of her, how her itchy and very uncomfortable throat had anything to do with a cold!

Have you noticed how your children never listen to anything you say but accept every word if it comes from their teachers? Or even anyone else? For instance, if I am teaching them Math, they are quick to tell me that's not what their teacher said…and of course, because their teacher can't be wrong, I am! 😃 But I digress…

So, it's that season, where everyone you see appears to be coughing or sniffling. If you have got children, you can try very hard, but you may not be able to avoid it…especially with everyone lovingly coughing and sneezing right into your face and nose. 😃

But we can encourage the virus not to move around much by doing the following:

85

- Wash your hands often and avoid touching your face as it helps spread the infection.

- A small tube of hand sanitizer is also useful for those times when you can't wash your hands.

- Drink lots of warm fluids. Soups are also not a bad idea during moments like this

- Cough into the crook of your arm and not into people's faces or private spaces. And of course, be sure to take a bath later in the day and wash those clothes too to get rid of the germs.

- If you use tissues at any point, please dispose of properly and then wash your hands…again. Be careful not to hurt the sides of your nose from frequent use of tissue for your leaky or runny nose.

- Some pain relief for your sore throat may come in handy but be sure not to take more than the recommended dose.

- Rest and help your body heal. While at it, remember to change your toothbrush after you have healed. This way, you won't re-infect yourself with germs you have kicked!

- And this may not be a great time to share love by sharing cups, toothbrushes and drinks.

Remember that you do not need antibiotics for a common cold. It is a viral infection which will run its course and leave the same way it came…uninvited.

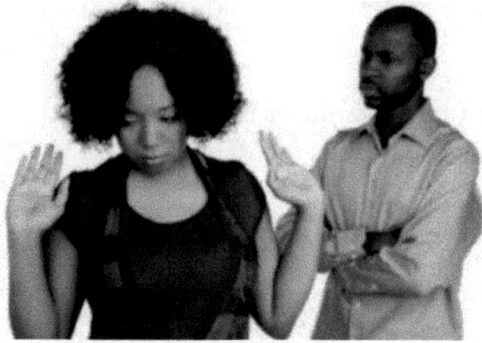

The Blame Game

It was children's day on the 27th of May, and I was at an event to give a talk on good hygiene to the kids. In the course of the event, I had cause to use the bathroom. It was absolutely atrocious what I saw there. Children using the bathroom in really terrible ways while their parents watched.

There were children urinating on the floor! In a bathroom that had modern conveniences, I could not find a toilet that was neat enough to be use; without water on the floor. Disgusting water in which millions and millions of germs were swimming and looking for another home.

As if that wasn't bad enough, as soon as they were done with the dirty deed, they all turned and walked right out of the bathroom. No hand washing…in fact, they were grabbed by the hands and shooed right out of the bathroom. Now this is doubly disgusting! First these children messed up a bathroom that (I assume) was perfectly clean when they came in. In the course of that, they got some germs on them and on their hands. Now without the hand washing, they were certified to go spread these germs to their friends waiting outside, through holding hands, sharing snacks or even just hugging.

I was in shock! Please parents, remember that your children's behaviour, attitude and health lie in your hands. If you don't teach them how to use the bathroom, how on earth will they learn? If you don't teach them how to wash their hands, or even how germs get into their bodies, how can they possibly prevent these germs from becoming a problem?

The shock I felt is the same one I feel when I observe people passing dirty places and spitting. My question is if you found that place disgusting, are you not making it doubly so for people who would pass after you? First they have to deal with the site of your spittle and then confront whatever it was that you saw or smelt in the first instance. Perhaps, this person (person 2) may decide to spit too, for good measure and then we create an unending cycle of filth and disease!

Studies had shown that a significant reduction in the presence of diseases in the world was observed when good sanitation became a way of life. So it wasn't totally because of the presence of vaccines and antibiotics rather, it was mainly due to good hygiene. In fact, especially in sub-Saharan Africa, respiratory infections and diarrheal diseases are known to be the greatest killers of under-5s. The reason is not farfetched; unwashed dirty hands used to prepare foods, causing diarrhoea or unwashed hands put into mouths by children, people sneezing into their hands and shaking people who in turn inhale these germs…the means of spreading these germs could go on and on.

To show how important simple hygienic practices are, studies have proved that in areas where hand washing was introduced, the incidence of diarrheal diseases and respiratory infections reduced by half. Let's add numbers to this to make it clearer: if there were twenty children out of one hundred dying every year from these infections, with the introduction of hand washing, this reduces to ten children. From hand washing alone!

This is basic knowledge, so how come, we still have children who mess up toilets while parents look on in approval? Who is to blame? The Government who hasn't provided an opportunity for this woman to be educated, so that she knows what is appropriate and what is not? The lack of 'in your face' health education programs to keep re-enforcing the hygiene message? The parent who should know better...if they have been given the opportunity? The children who go to school and have been taught to wash their hands after using the bathroom (we hope) and yet choose not to practice same? Or perhaps at every point that these lessons ought to have been taught, people looked the other way and felt it wasn't their problem. That means it's our collective fault.

We can rectify it today. Teach a child how and when to wash their hands. Teach them to sneeze into the crooks of their elbows and not their hands. Teach them to wash their hands for at least twenty seconds. Teach them to rub the soap their hands properly and teach them to rinse their hands well.

Remember that an ounce of protection is better than a pound of cure...or in popular parlance, prevention is better than cure.

You Are What You Read

If we were to take this title literally, what would you be? Should we attempt to give names to people based on what they read? Hmm, interesting thought…but we probably won't get to the business of the day! So, reluctantly, I give this up!

I love travelling. No, let me amend that. I love the freedom I have when I travel. On the flight, I know that for the number of hours it takes me to get to my destination, I am very unlikely to be disturbed with a phone call. (By the way, can someone tell the airlines that it is not a cool idea to enable phone calls while in the air? I'm not sure whether this has finally been done or whether it is still a plan. Either way, please someone let them know what I think. I don't want anyone to get in touch with me while I am in the air. That's me time! 😃).

I love the fact that when I check into my hotel or wherever, I don't have to make dinner or worry about breakfast, etc. I can decide to eat or not. But the very best part of all this is what I have saved for last. This is when I catchup on all my reading…and please note that I don't mean heavy duty reading. Very light, fun-filled easy on the eyes reading. I touch base with John Grisham and his humour that keeps me doubled over in laughter, the suspense of Fredrick Forsyth's novels, the intrigue of Jeffrey Archer's characters, etc. I read, I sleep and then of course, I attend to the business that brought me there. But I just love the freedom to read a novel.

Friends who know me from way back always ask me whether I still read novels as much as I did back then. I would read novels even when I was supposed to be preparing for examinations. That was my way of unwinding after tedious reading and this habit followed me all the way to the university (By the way, note that this is not a recipe for success. Actually, it is a recipe for disaster, and I issue the immediate disclaimer that nobody should be found reading a novel while preparing for exams! 😃) I don't read that many novels anymore. I now have too many things pulling at me!

I started off with Ladybirds. We had a whole library filled with all the classics… Snow white (with the Seven Dwarfs and with Rose Red), Sleeping Beauty, Goldilocks, etc. Then I moved on to Pacesetters. These novels introduced me to the world of adult reading. It was a mixed grill of action, suspense and romance. Ah, romance. What Pacesetters introduced, Mills and Boon took to a whole new level; I would like to ask a question though, 'has anyone ever seen 'that' tall, dark and handsome chap (rich to boot of course)' that we all read about in our M & B's? If you see him, summon him into my presence. 😃

Back to our gist. This is not about me or my good or bad reading habits. It is about this habit in our children. Children do not just read anymore. There are a 'gazillion' things pulling at them, but reading…novels or anything is not one of those things. And it is not just here…it's everywhere.

My children and I took a quick vacation and on one of our outings; all three of them had a book in their faces. When they said hello to a lady in the elevator with us, she actually commented that it is so good to see children reading. That made my heart glow. I mean I would love to tell you that I have got these perfect children who read all the time and don't have to be reminded. I really wish I could tell you that. 😄 But the truth is that, it is not that way. My first daughter would fall into that category (I saw her attempting to read a novel while taking a bath once. That settled it! I had to ban reading from certain activities 😊). For the other two, it is carrot and stick approach. You have your daily chores for a week and then you have also to read a book during that week. If you do your chores satisfactorily, there is an allowance at the end of the week and then if a book was successfully finished, there is an additional little something. Am I bribing these children to read? I try not to think of it in that sense. I like to think that I am encouraging a good habit in them…and, by the way, during that holiday, they did not get any allowance for chores or anything else. So I must be succeeding in encouraging this habit…I think. 😊

We are bringing up a generation of children who do not read, cannot write in complete sentences and are too lazy to reason through an issue when they can google it. I am sure my children think I am a pain when I insist that text messages must be written in long hand. I mean, let's face it. Letters are so last year (so they tell me) that beyond marking their English comprehension work (if you do), the only written correspondence you are ever likely to have on a continuous basis with your children are text messages and perhaps e-mails. So they had better be good!

Reading also teaches them to 'travel' the world and visit other cultures and indeed learn to appreciate other cultures, people, traditions and religions. It develops their imaginations and gets them to; hopefully, think out of the box. Let's have some more Einsteins please; people who will redefine the face of the earth, thinkers who will go after their dreams rather than expect them to be handed to them on a platter of gold, readers who are leaders and who will birth the next generation of readers. When you read, you have a rich store of words that are useful in different circumstances. Let's stop having those...emmm, what's the right word to use?...moments (I am guilty too...sometimes!)

We, the parents are no better. We only read fashion magazines and the gossip rags. Before you look for the rotten tomatoes to pelt me with, please note that I am not averse to a good gossip now and again, but we really have to feed our brains.

Read management books, or self-development books or even novels. Or newspapers...what's up with PDP, new or old? What's happening in Jos? Iran? Syria? Beyond being good conversation starters, it shows how knowledgeable you are and generally improves mental health. It is disheartening especially when young people come in for job interviews and have no idea of topical issues; some cannot even tell you anything about the company they profess to want to work for! It is mind boggling. There is just no quest for knowledge or excellence.

We can actually inculcate this love for reading in children very early by reading to them when they are very young. As you tuck them into bed, and they say their prayers, then settle in for a short or long read to them. This encourages bonding with your children, creates an intimate time when they know they can ask you any question, they develop longer attention span and indeed logical reasoning.

So lead by example and create a reading time for the whole family...you know, the same way you all gather to watch TV? And if you are not married, read too. It's never too late to start a good habit. Feed your mind and build your mental health.

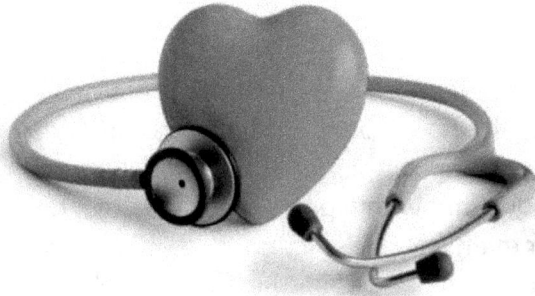

The Gateway To The Heart!

How come you feel sad or cry when a sad song is played? Think about it…that's right. It's because you heard the lyrics and perhaps it tugged at a memory. What about the pain you feel when that person you care about hurls some really nasty words at you? It is almost like your heart is going to break, right?

All these emotions can be experienced through one gateway only…the ears!

Have you ever wondered whether you are taking good care of your ears? Weird question, right? Like, what can go wrong with your ears? They generally mind their business on the sides of our heads and more often than not, we don't even notice them. That is kind of why when you take the pain to look behind them, especially for children, you find 'amazing' stuff there…disgustingly smelly stuff, that much I can tell you!

Well, I never used to pay much mind to these hearing organs until I had children. One weekend, my first daughter gingerly walked into my room and complained about a funny sensation in her ears. I probed about whether this was water in the ear, an itch, a buzzing sound…what? I decided to look in. What did I see…? a pencil tip! No! How on earth does something on a writing instrument end up in the ear? How did this happen? How…? The questions were popping out faster than I could ask them.

The story came out…pretty basic and simple story, really. She felt an itch in her ear; she had a pencil in her hand and generally scratched the itch with it. Pretty simple really…you feel an itch, you scratch it. Yes? Well yes, just not with a pencil or sharp object…especially when it's your ear or even eye. So, we ended up in the ENT (Ear, Nose and Throat) doctor's office where the 'foreign object' was removed. Thankfully no lasting damage had been done to her ear drum or any other part of the ear.

Next episode came via my second daughter who anytime she swam kept us awake the whole night screaming about her ears! I almost considered banning swimming as her case of Swimmer's ears was always more than I could bear.
What is Swimmer's ears, I hear you ask? This usually occurs when the outer ear becomes moist and warm from frequent swimming. The natural oily, waxy protection of the ear canal is also washed away. Thus, bacteria have the ideal environment (warm and moist) to thrive in and can do so without any fear of being trapped by the wax that has been washed away. This condition would usually start off with tingling or itching in the ear…you know the type; you can't resist scratching 😊 … but try to resist it, as this just worsens a bad situation by breaking the delicate skin of your ear, letting in even more bacteria! Other times, this condition would show up as pain in the ear with some discharge too.

The final ear episode I remember also started with ear pain or itch. We ended up in the ENT doctor's office again this time for removal of impacted wax.

Now, what's the moral in these stories? There is something to be said for caring for our ears. For instance, our common practice of cleaning our ears with cotton tips or cotton buds should be discouraged. These actually push wax deeper into the ears. They can also harm the delicate lining of your ear and in extreme cases; bore a hole in your ear drum! In fact, conventional wisdom states that we should not clean our ears with anything bigger than our elbows....uh huh! You heard me...your elbows! So, just wash your outer ears with a washcloth while taking a bath...this is more than sufficient cleaning!

Other tips to take care of your ears when swimming:

- Choose clean pools or waters to swim in.
- Use a swimming cap and use it to shield your ears.
- It is probably inevitable that some water will get into your ears, but don't just let it sit there. Shake it out.

The wax actually serves a purpose...to trap foreign objects that may want to go deeper down into your ears and cause damage. So, leave it alone to get on with this job.

Constantly using earphones may also lead to problems in your ear...recall how it appears your ears feel inflamed after a while?

Remember that pencils, pens or their covers are not meant to be used to scratch your ear or remove wax. If you do find a foreign body in your ear, don't try to get anyone to fish it out, see your doctor!

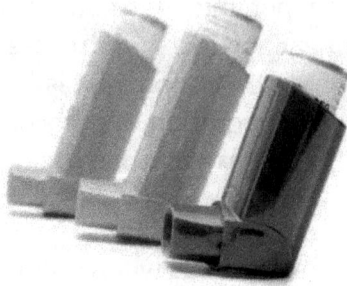

Asthma

Asthma is a disease that affects quite a few in our population. If you are a mother with an asthmatic child, you will remember the heart wrenching agony you felt when the diagnosis was first given to you. You imagined a lifetime of wheezing and crises. However, this may not be so. Hygiene around the house plays a large role in ensuring that allergens which are substances that provoke allergies and could start up an asthmatic attack are on the low side. Therefore, your stays child healthy.

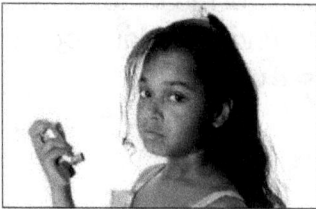

Dust mites are small organisms that are not visible to the naked eyes and found in fabric, feathers and wool. Thus, they are usually resident in pillows and feed on dead skin that human beings shed normally everyday. They love moisture and heat and so can be found on beds. As a result, of the sweat from people. Though they do not fly, as beds are being made they can fly across the room and cause allergic reactions on people who are prone or trigger an asthmatic attack in people with these conditions.

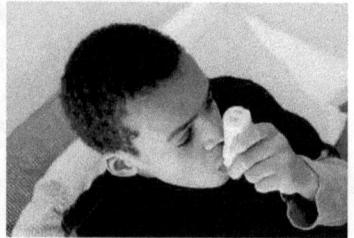

How to hold this small but mighty organism at bay? Here are our top five tips;

- Remove dust. Try dusting with a damp napkin or an oiled duster. This ensures that the dust doesn't get airborne to settle somewhere else; worse still to settle inside the airways of an asthmatic. This is sure to provoke an attack. Try vacuuming instead of using a broom or brush.

- Use allergen-proof mattress covers. These covers are tightly woven; they trap and prevent the dust mites from escaping from the mattress to provoke the airways into spasm.

- Wash bedding every week. This should also be done for stuffed toys. Ensure that this is done with hot water to kill the dust mites and remove allergens. And stuffed toys should be kept off bedding.

- Limit the use of carpeting and other dust collecting items of furniture around the house like curtains and upholstered chairs. These are major reservoirs of dust mites. Scrub, polish and keep your floors clean; change curtains to horizontal blinds and reduce the population of these mites significantly.

- Keep the moisture and humidity low and reduce clutter. These would reduce the breeding places of the mites.

With simple hygiene tips, even diseases like asthma can be controlled. So join us as we do this.

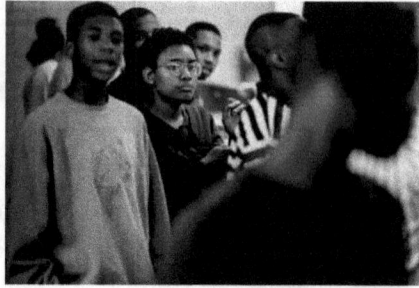

Adolescence... 10 Going On 30!

My first daughter turned 11 recently. Remember the one that I made a princess during her first school party? The very same one is 11! Where did all that time fly to? Not too long ago, I was changing her diapers and weaning her and teaching her to eat by herself and now she is all grown up... and actually has the temerity to call me her daughter sometimes! Yeah, she is taller than I am, but... the cheek of her! 😃

With her adolescence, though, come some very difficult issues to tackle like sex education and other delicate matters. I mean, why do I want to discuss that stuff with my little daughter? When she was younger, it was easier to 'avoid' these conversations as I could just buy nicely worded and beautifully coloured books that talk about HIV/AIDS and STI's and leave it at that. A few awkward questions and we're all good to go. But I can't hide behind the books anymore. This is the time for face to face, 'I-want-to-know-how-it-works' and sometimes, despite the brave smile on my face, I cringe inwardly about what we are discussing!

However, the statistics provide enough incentive not to give up and to keep conversation lines open. Did you know that the World Health Organization estimates that 16 million adolescent girls (young people aged between ten and nineteen years) give birth every year, and most of them are in low and middle income countries (just in case you wondered, Nigeria is certainly one of these!). These girls, especially those in the fifteen to nineteen age bracket, are more likely to die from the complications of pregnancy and childbirth…and the terrible statistics continue.

This is about the age when adolescents discover alcohol and other drugs…perhaps by watching television, other adults, peers or even the internet. And this is the time they try their hands at experimenting with this stuff. An adolescent under the influence of alcohol or indeed any other drug is more likely to make bad decisions about sex, than a sober one, thus complicating an already bad scenario.

This is the time for frank and open conversations. Do you recall when we were younger (that's if you're in my age group 😊) and some parents would tell their children that if a guy looked at them, they would get pregnant? Forget those old wives' tales. They are not relevant today because these children probably know the names of things that you didn't even know existed…maybe. So be open about the issues that you are concerned about and find out what your adolescent thinks about those issues…in as open and non-judgemental way as possible. If you can get into their heads, you have got a better chance of figuring out what's going on there and perhaps, tightening any loose screws. 😊

Make out time to do stuff with them. I know we all get busy with work and other activities, but the children really need positive mentors at this stage. Statistics show that children who spend more time with their parents and are involved with activities generally stay out of trouble more. Remember the saying, an idle mind is the devil's workshop? Let them discover activities they are really good at: arts and crafts, sports or singing and get them involved in organizations that encourage these.

I am very old school about social media with regards to my children. Even the websites realise that there are specific ages at which these 'children' should be given the liberty to associate with people they don't even know, and that's why they have age limits. Stick with those and even then, discuss the positives and negatives of these new media. They have to be careful who they are friending, befriending, unfriending, whatsapping, tweeting, 'wechatting' and emailing!

I had an interesting discussion about a week ago with some researchers from out of town (United States) who came to research teenage pregnancy and Termination Of Pregnancies (TOPs). I wasn't of much help though I pointed them in the direction of some Government centers, first because TOPs are illegal in Nigeria and secondly because the only information that might exist may be in the Government approved centres. But they asked me a curious question before they left, "if a teenager you knew got pregnant, what would you have them do: abort the baby or keep the baby given their absolute lack of preparedness to deal with a baby?"

Tough one… and in very typical Nigerian fashion, my first thought was 'I reject it in Jesus' name!' Suffice it to say that my answer was long winded and convoluted and probably ended up giving me a headache! My head still throbs when I think of it. 😊

More seriously though, it is a wake-up call to everyone who has teenagers or mentors teenagers to face these issues head on and provide the right information. Focus on short term and medium term consequences as opposed to long term ones. It is usually difficult for a teenager to look far enough into the future to figure out how a pregnancy now messes with their ability get a good job later and fend for their family adequately. This has multiple rebound effects on their own children who will probably not be able to meet their own potentials later in life.

Focus on them not being able to go to the prom or gain admission into the university…that can't very well happen when they've got a baby to look after, right? How they will disappoint a mentor that they are particularly fond of and how most importantly, they will be devaluing their sense of self-worth.

As we keep having these discussions, hopefully we can help reduce the statistics and have a more productive generation.

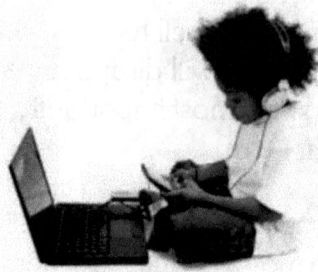

Tough Love And Generation Z

The good old days! It is just mind boggling for me whenever I realize that I've known some people for more than twenty years! Whhaaaat!!! Am I that old? I still remember the shock on my face and the way I looked around in confusion the first day someone referred to me as 'Ma. 'Who, me!?! But I am certainly no spring chicken anymore (sob, sob). I belong to the generation when Television Stations started by 4.00 pm and before they did, we all excitedly gazed at the colour bars on our television sets waiting for them to start the day's business (assuming you had adequately done your homework).

Beyond televisions, there were the VHS video machines which our parents may allow us to turn on at the weekends…again, only if homework and house chores had been completed. The only other source of distraction which was acceptable to our parents and could be practiced at all times was reading. As a child, I read voraciously starting from ladybirds to Pacesetters and yes, Mills and Boon! Uh!! That tall, handsome and rich guy who was to come sweep me off

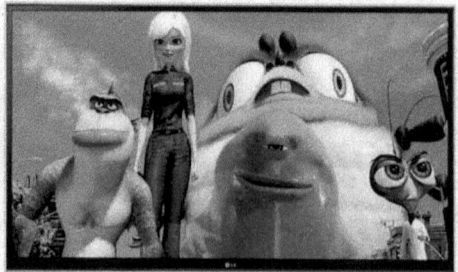

my feet!!! From there, I moved on and explored other worlds of books and eventually arrived at the stables of John Grisham…the master story teller, with wit, sarcasm and suspense. Till today, I find myself screaming with laughter whenever I read any of his novels. My driver always steals surreptitious glances through the rear view mirror…almost as if he were wondering when it would be appropriate to scream for help (Help! My boss has gone crazy!).

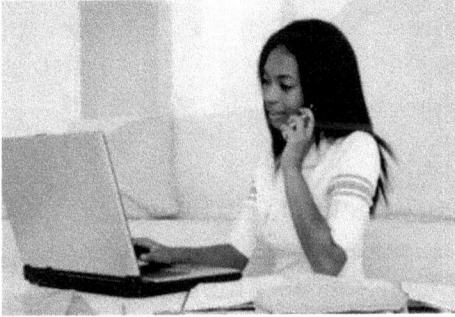

Speaking of novels, have you ever wondered how many children we see these days reading a book? They absolutely hate the idea, not with television on from the morning till forever, with all manner of programs, alongside newer and 'better' video games coming out every single day.

These children are well versed in spoken English but cannot correctly write down the grammar they so eloquently speak. They do not know synonyms, antonyms, verbs, nouns, adjectives, collective nouns and all those stuff they made us learn (and boy, did you have to learn?!) every single day. These children have lost…scratch that…never even had the opportunity to learn logical reasoning. And so, we are bringing up children who are intellectually and mentally lazy; unable to think for themselves and certainly not able to think outside the box.

Now, before you all (or maybe some of you) crucify me for being a party pooper, let me explain that I love the Generation Z children (can we shorten this to Gen Zeezers…just thinking); those children born between 1995 and 2012…I mean, I really have no choice. I have three of them, and I love them to bits! I also do not have anything against these games, and I certainly love my TV shows over the weekends. BUT, these activities should not become the focal point of our existence. Younger mothers 'plop' their children down before the television as a babysitting ploy.

Our children are beginning to find it difficult to think for themselves, reason a problem all the way through or even make an effort to reflect on anything. They want quick answers, and they want it now. They get it from the internet…which is a good thing, but they have got to be able to even think about the issues they want to research before getting the easy answers.

The problem has moved beyond the home to the workplace. You interview tens to find one employee and hundreds to find ten. These young men and women cannot answer the most mundane of questions and sometimes, look around almost like they are looking for hints from somewhere.

What is the solution? Let us get these children busy with other stuff. They have to read a book for at least two hours every day; where they fail that, withdraw some privileges…and don't let the puppy dog face fool you!

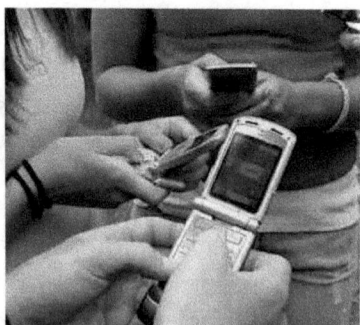

When they come to you with a problem, get them to think it through and try to figure out a solution before you even offer an opinion; homework and projects are meant to be done by them. You are only to provide strategic support in terms of asking questions that lead them to question what they have done. We used to play a game when we were young, where we would have a very long word, and the contest was to find the person who would make the most words out of that long word. This helped us think of all the words in there and better still, we never looked at a word ordinarily anymore. We were always trying to figure out how many words could be formed from any word we saw...long or short. It was fun, and it is still fun today...at least my children 'pretend' to enjoy it...path of least resistance, I guess. 😄

Remember to try and explain the reasons for these activities you have planned for them. As cool as it is (I think) to say, 'just because mummy or daddy said so!' It is probably better and helps with building their mental health to explain the benefits of what you are asking them to do. They probably would want to do it without much persuasion subsequently. And, this is a different generation from ours when we did 'exactly' as we were told without asking questions....I'm still trying to figure out if this is a good change or not. Oh, the good old days... What do you think?

Get children to play scrabble...in fact play with them. It builds their vocabulary...even those crazy, I-don't know-what-they-mean words! Get them to play monopoly...it teaches them the rudiments of financial management and don't be too quick to solve life's problems for them. They need to learn that life is full of curves and be prepared to handle what life throws at them. This is called tough love and builds mental health as well as develops their character. We see so many people today who stand for nothing...a man has to stand for something!

Remember that the more time they spend in front of the television or playing all those games, the less time they also spend outside...playing football, riding bikes, chasing after each other, playing lawn tennis, skipping, etc. In fact, several studies have linked excessive television watching and by extension playing with all those handheld computer games with a high incidence of obesity and the resulting medical conditions that go with that including Diabetes and Hypertension. This has to stop.

Imagine a child who is born into a family of Hypertensive and already has to deal with the burden of knowing that he is pre-disposed to the illness, living a lifestyle that clearly pushes him to that condition. He could have side-stepped this if we, as parents, make the right moves to get them to do the right thing. Please note that playing outside is also a function of neighbourhoods: If safe, pull out all the stops. If not, find other means of getting them to exercise…maybe enrolling in a swimming class in a club, dancing class, organizing play dates with their friends that live in safer neighbourhoods, etc.

Please note that children should actually be making about twelve thousand footsteps per day. Do I see you nodding your head and assuming that they must rack this up? Especially with all the activities they manage to invent per day? Or when they get to school? Get them pedometers…the result will shock you. They don't!

We need to do something people, to improve our children's mental and physical health by giving them more recreational activities than television and game consoles. Let's safeguard the next generation. They will thank you for it at some point in their lives. I once came across the saying, 'by the time you are old enough to know your parents were right, you probably have children who think you are wrong!' So, maybe not today, but…sometime in the very fuzzy future, there will be an 'Aha' moment and you will be glad, you made that happen.

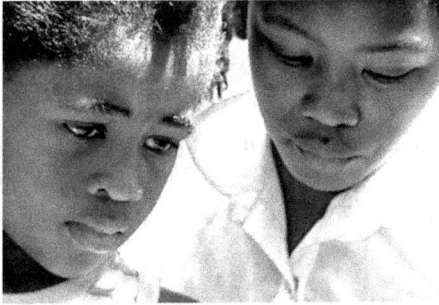

Hang tough... dont puff!

When I was younger, the picture of a cool guy wasn't complete without a cigarette in his hands. Then, if he had a cigar, men, that was hyper-ultra-cool! He would usually be seen leaning on a cool car, with lots of other dudes hanging on to his words and pretty girls dying to be given the eye by him. In fact, some television adverts for cigarettes would go so far as to show how with puffs of cigarettes, a regular guy not only becomes super-cool but also becomes a super athlete, star, etc. Do they actually possess these powers? Hmmm!

It was World No Tobacco day a while ago. It really went by quietly, with not much noise. I think I just caught a tiny paragraph in the newspaper where a company executive from one of the tobacco companies talked about how much they were doing in terms of corporate social responsibility. The focus for this year's celebration was banning tobacco advertising: 'Ban tobacco advertising, sponsorship and promotion.'

The tobacco companies, to be fair to them, actually note on the packs that smokers are likely to die young. But I have always thought the adverts were not really telling us anything. Die from what exactly? People who cross the roads without looking are likely to die young;

people who do not use the pedestrian crossings and instead choose to cross the expressway are likely to die young, any person who falls in front of a fast moving train will most certainly die, young or old. In fact, my friends delight in telling me whenever I sound sanctimonious that 'na something go kill person.' These are the adult, almost 'ossified' fossils like me.

For the younger ones, repercussions that are too far in the future are difficult to comprehend today when they are all hip and cool. The talk of all the consequences is kinda like lots of smoke without fire! And the tobacco companies have also gotten innovative; they take the advert to where the young ones actually hang out. The time of discovering tobacco is about the same time that alcohol is discovered and so the young ones are hanging around bars and night clubs (I thought there were age limits for admission.).This is where the tobacco companies go, and they have a huge and captive audience.

Tobacco use has a lot of health implications and has been noted as a risk factor in lung diseases, heart diseases and cancers. This may appear to be too far in the future and difficult for our teenagers who are in their prime to contemplate. So, perhaps educating them about more short to medium term consequences may be helpful. Some of these include:

- Reduced fitness levels…making them appear old and fuddy-duddy! They can't even join the cool sports teams.

- Nasty smelling breath that even toothpaste, breath mints and candy cannot mask.

- Becoming unattractive to non-smoking peers

- Stained teeth and fingers

- Wasting money that could be used for clothes, music or other items

- Finally, the fact that the teenager loses control and can't stop smoking once addiction to nicotine appears.

I had a very close relation who smoked...a lot. He also drank...a lot. He eventually died with complications of hypertension, Diabetes Mellitus, liver cirrhosis and lung disease. Granted, there was a whole lot more going on than just the smoking but it's now a case of which came first, 'the cart or the horse.' I don't know, but I can surely tell you that smoking didn't help him any.

Tobacco use is a major preventable cause of death worldwide. The reasons for tobacco use are many and diverse, but in a nutshell, appears to be a way from which people attempt to escape the stress and the pressures of life. So the campaign for eradicating smoking goes beyond the individual and involves the Government which must provide the right socio-economic support for the issues people stress out about. Having said that, we also have a role to play.

For adult smokers, there has to be a clear desire to quit and so being positive, being around supportive people and avoiding the areas where one usually is encouraged to smoke, are steps in the right direction. Getting other hobbies, switching to oral substitutes like chewing gum, carrots and mints are also helpful. Brushing your teeth often is also a good idea as toothpaste makes cigarette taste really bad...so I hear.

Methinks though that the best way to discourage your teenagers from smoking is by setting a good example. They learn much more from what we do than from what we say.

So guys, I say, 'let's tar our roads, not our lungs!'

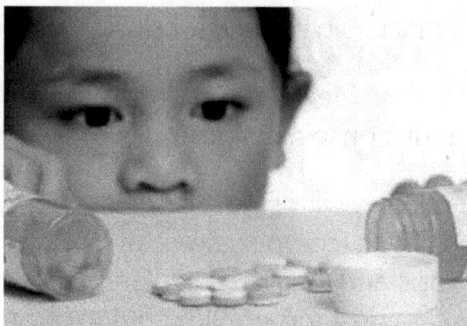

Substance Abuse

Substance abuse is becoming a major problem in our environment as teenagers move from the stages of experimentation to total dependence on these drugs.
Here are five ways to help your children avoid substance abuse:

Spend time with them. We all get too busy with one thing or the other and do not spend quality time with our teens. Teens with hands-on parents who are involved in their lives are more likely to avoid drugs and alcohol. Families that spend time together, hang out and eat meals together have more opportunities for insightful and continual conversation. Discuss ways for your child to make responsible choices, no matter what his or her friends are saying or doing. Praise achievements. Never miss a chance to praise your child and build his or her self-esteem.

Encourage them to join a team. Sports build self-esteem. Studies have shown that teenagers involved with sports are less likely to get involved with drugs or alcohol as teammates and coaches have expectations for everyone on the team to be playing to their full potential. Most teams also apply strict sobriety rules, which create a huge incentive for teens to stay clean.

Get them involved with an organization of interest. If sports is not your teenager's thing, get him involved in some other extra-curricular activity; arts, music or spiritual groups. These help keep the teenagers busy and interacting with groups that build a sense of positive self-worth.

Be open and have discussions about drug abuse and consequences. Forget the old wives' tales we were told as children about the consequences of drugs. Focus on facts and get them involved in figuring out how to avoid peer pressure when drugs are offered. Remember that even a teenager can develop a drug problem.

Ask your teen's opinion. Listen to your teenager's opinion on the issue. Watch the body language and do not be judgmental. If they sense this, they can clam up, and you will be none the wiser as to their real views on drug use or whether they are using drugs already.

Beyond all these, Show good example. Teenagers learn a lot more from what we do than what we say!

QUESTIONS And Answers

WHY IS MY BABY'S TUMMY RUMBLING?

Q: Please, what do you think can be causing my baby's tummy to make sounds and what can be done to prevent this?

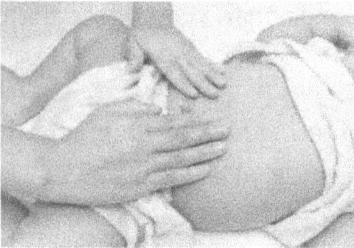

A: Your baby's tummy makes noise normally...grumbling noises, murmuring noises, gurgling noises, etc. all through the day and they are normal. You would probably notice them more just before your baby eats or soon after. Those are the sounds of our very hard working intestines as they contract and push air around i.e. swallowed air and air produced as a result, of digestion.

As long as your baby eats normally, does not have abdominal pain and is not vomiting, then there is probably no problem. These sounds are very loud and active just after a meal or when your child eats foods like beans.

The normal process of digesting beans involves fermentation in the intestines which, of course, produces more gas and by extension, more bowel sounds. When one has diarrhea, these sounds happen more frequently and conversely, reduce when one is constipated.

In fact, little or no bowel sounds after a meal may be suggestive of a problem. In the same way, very high pitched sounds could also mean there are issues. You would, of course, need to know what the normal sound is in order to recognise the strange sounds. As I always say, when in doubt, please consult your doctor.

HELP! MY CHILD IS LOSING ALL HER HAIR!

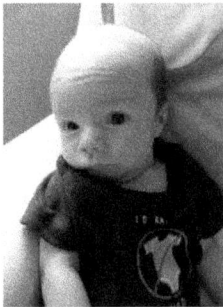

Q: Doctor, I am a little worried about my daughter's hair. She is two months-plus and was born very hairy, but now all her hair seems to be pulling out. Please, what can I use to stop this because I am really worried?

A: Within the first six months of life, a baby may lose quite a bit of hair due mainly to a reduction in certain hormone levels. In fact, some lose quite a lot of hair, and when it grows back, it has a different texture and sometimes, even colour! If your baby also has a specific way of lying down, perhaps on her back, you may notice thinning of the hair in that area.   So, do not worry! When in doubt, however, please see your doctor who will take a look and confirm whether you have something to worry about.

IS MY BABY TEETHING TOO EARLY?

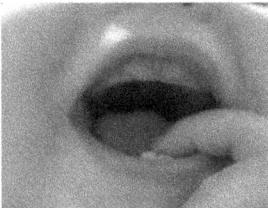

Q: My son is just three months, but he already has three teeth. People say it's too early. How true is this?

A: Your baby is certainly in a hurry. 🙂 Seriously though, babies start teething at different times. On the average, most children start teething at six months. Some start earlier than 4 months (as early as two months) and some others may wait up to a year or even after, to start the journey. Some children are even born with one or two teeth. These are called natal teeth and 'No, this is not associated with witchcraft or enemies pressing remote controls' as we like to think in Africa. 😊

Some children also develop their own teeth within the first four weeks of life. These are called neonatal teeth. Natal and neonatal teeth can cause problems with feeding and may even be swallowed. The paediatric dentist will decide whether to remove them or leave them alone based on factors like whether the teeth are loose, excess, etc.
Generally though, in instances like the one addressed in the question, provided the teeth do not negatively affect baby's feeding, they should be left alone.

I THINK MY DAUGHTER IS SMALL FOR HER AGE!

Q: My two year old daughter doesn't add body weight, and she doesn't like eating. Sometimes she eats very well and at other times she does not. She is also small for her age. What should I do?

A: Hmm! I'm sure every mum has heard this and has this fear! In fact, my second daughter was a major challenge for me. She was tiny and refused to eat anything…literally She constantly had her baby cup in her mouth and essentially lived on a fluid diet at a time when her mates were eating 'major' food! I kept begging God not to let her be malnourished…what would I tell people? 😊
But guess what? She appears to be making up for lost ground…eating everything in sight. Thankfully too, she does love to eat healthy…the only one of my children I really don't have to force….or to be more polite, encourage to eat right.

Remember that children, like all of us, are creatures of comfort and habit. So we really don't want any change in what we are used to eating. This is especially more so for a two year old. If you have let her 'dictate' to a large extent what she eats and what she does not up till this age, then it is a bit more difficult at this moment to 'regiment' her feeding habits than when she was a year old 😊 However, that doesn't mean that it can't be done.
Here is what to do.

First, I try to remind parents that there's only one boss, and that's you! 😊 Your baby needs to understand that. And so, while your job is to provide a variety of foods for your baby to choose from (as best you can), it is your baby's job to pick from these.

Therefore, if you provide two options of either brown rice with sardine sauce and steamed vegetables or Amala with Ewedu, stew and chicken for lunch, the choice she gets is which one of these she wants; rice or amala. 😊

This, of course, is for a start as you try to tempt and encourage her taste buds to try different things (I can see a lot of you already asking, 'am I going to prepare two lunches every time?'. The answer is No 😊).

Try to prepare balanced meals with foods from all food groups and try different (healthy) ways of preparing them. Introduce fruits and vegetables early so that this habit is formed early and they grow up seeing that, eating with a plate half-filled with veggies, with the other half shared between carbs and protein, is normal. 😊 Try different things until you discover the right combination.

A lot of times, because we are all busy with stuff, it's convenient to make quick noodles and give cookies and then complain that it's all the baby eats. However, when was the last time you made the effort to prepare something else and really encourage the baby to eat? Weaning or introduction of complementary feeds is not an easy task for most parents, and it does require effort…a lot of it!

To confirm that your child is not adding any weight at all, and this pre-supposes that you weigh her regularly do a quick calculation of your baby's ideal weight from ages 1 year to 5 years, multiply her age in years by 2 and add 8 $(2n + 8)$.

From our calculations, your baby's ideal weight should be about 12kg. But this poses another question. Is she adding weight monthly but perhaps not as much as expected? Not gaining weight at all, is a major health issue that actually goes beyond eating. If she adds weight but not up to what is expected, the problem may be with not getting enough nutrients, either in quality or quantity. Please see her paediatrician to ensure you are not just being overly anxious as all mothers worldwide, from the beginning of time, are known to be. ☺

Remember that to help the process of growth, your baby should get enough sleep (especially an afternoon nap) and some exercise and playtime (at least 30 minutes per day).

MY BABY HAS KNOCK-KNEES (K LEGS). WHAT SHOULD I DO?

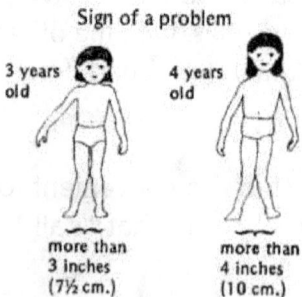

Sign of a problem

3 years old

4 years old

more than 3 inches (7½ cm.)

more than 4 inches (10 cm.)

Q: Please Doctor, what of knock knees? My son who is two years and five months suddenly developed knock-knees when he was a year and eight months. Please, what can I do about it? Please, help me because I am very worried.

A: Knock-knees (or K legs, as we call them in these parts) may not necessarily be a cause for alarm. From birth to eighteen months, baby's legs tend to bend in a bow fashion. When this is not due to disease (Blount's disease or rickets), it is usually due to their position in the womb and corrects normally.

From 18 months to 24 months, the legs go into neutral mode. Not much happening, one way to the other but from two years to five years of age, knock-knees take center stage and would usually increase in severity until about 4 years of age.

When children with knock-knees stand, their knees touch but their ankles don't. Usually, this corrects spontaneously around six to seven years of age, and if it doesn't, can be corrected with braces. If knock knees appear for the first time by the age of six years, it may be due to a disease condition.

In situations that do not self-correct and are not amenable to braces, surgery may be the other option.

So, this is also treatable 😊

WHAT CAN I DO ABOUT THESE BOW LEGS?

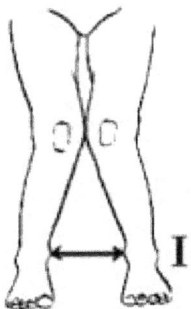

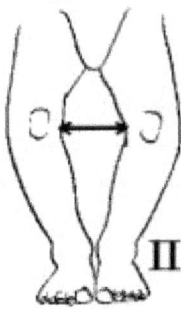

Q: I have a sister who is 16 years that is bow-legged. Is there any drug she can take that doesn't involve surgical attention that she can take?

A: Bowlegs (genu varum) would usually occur in children when they are born because of the position they adopt in the uterus (physiological bowing). This, however, would usually resolve and disappear without any treatment by the time they are 3 years old. However, in very few instances they do not resolve. Two other conditions Blount's disease and Rickets can lead to bow legs. In Blount's disease, there is an abnormality in the upper part of the shinbone (tibia) and in Rickets, the body is unable to absorb Vitamin D adequaetely or there is a lack of Vitamin D, calcium or phosphorus in the food taken by the baby.

When people with bow legs stand with their feet together, their knees do not touch, and there is an obvious bowing of the legs to the eyes.

For a child less than two years old with the same degree of bowing on both legs (symmetrical bowing), your doctor may not suggest more tests. This is likely to be physiological bowing. However, if the bowing is more on one side, then X-rays may reveal Blount's disease or Rickets.

Symmetrical bowing beyond age three years is unlikely to be physiological and is also suggestive of Blount's Disease or Rickets.

If physiological bowing continues into adolescence, surgery is the treatment of choice. If bowing is due to Blount's disease, braces can be used to correct this if noticed early. If not, again surgery is the fall back choice of treatment. If Rickets, however, is the bad guy, treatment can be commenced with replacement of deficient minerals (Vitamin D), and if this fails to correct it, surgery is done.

So, for your sister, it appears surgery may be the way to go if other treatment options noted are not applicable. Please ensure that she is seeing an orthopaedic surgeon who may also invite other specialists into the management, if need be.

So, now you know that if you have a bow-legged child, you can absolutely do something about it. Bowlegs are a major source of knee pain as one gets older. You don't want to subject your child to that later.

Ensure that your children get adequate amounts of sunshine daily and also be sure that you give foods that are fortified with Vitamin D.

WHAT CAN I DO TO HELP MY BABY WHO HAS CEREBRAL PALSY (CP)?

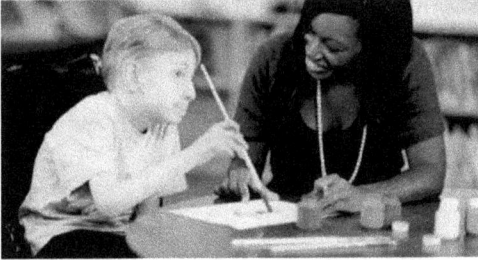

Q: Hello Doctor, my baby has CP, and I need your advice on how and when you think my baby can walk and live a normal life like every other child? Thanks.

A: Cerebral palsy (CP) is a disorder in which there are problems with movement, muscle tone and or posture that is caused by damage to baby's brain before, during or after birth during the first 3 to 5 years.

The signs and symptoms of this show up during infancy or the pre-school age and are dependent on the type of CP.

- Children with spastic CP experience difficulties with moving and stiffness
- Children with ataxic CP experience problems with their perception of depth and balance.
- Children with athetoid CP, experience involuntary and uncontrolled movements

Other problems that could be experienced by CP children include blindness, deafness, problems with swallowing and speaking, behavioural problems, tremors and epilepsy.

The precise causes of CP are not really known but pre-disposing factors include:

During pregnancy - damage or lack of proper development of the brain which may be due to infections (chicken pox, German measles, syphilis, exposure to toxins etc.) or genetic problems.

During labour and delivery - difficult labour and delivery which may lead to reduced oxygen supply to baby's brain (asphyxia)

Infections in a newly born baby - infections of the coverings of the brain or untreated jaundice.

Other conditions associated with CP include prematurity, multiple births, low-birth weight, malnutrition, car accidents in which babies were not properly restrained (by using car seats and suitable restraints) as well as shaking the baby in infancy, etc.

Unfortunately, there is no cure for CP, but, you can absolutely work with your child's team of medics to ensure that your child leads a normal life. Different types of therapies aimed at the different areas of challenges (movement, speech, learning, social and emotional development) especially if started early, are very helpful. Please ensure that your baby is getting all of these.

To prevent probable CP in children, be sure to take care of yourself during pregnancy, attend antenatal classes and take any needed medications and vaccinations, ensure that you use seat restraints (car-seat belts, baby-carriages with their restraints, etc.) when you have children in a car.

And finally, never give up! Keep doing everything you can and prayerfully encourage your baby even when it is frustrating. There is light at the end of the tunnel. Read avidly about any and everything available and don't be afraid to ask your baby's doctors question about any aspect of his or her care.

REAL OR ARTIFICIAL FEVER?

Q: Hello Doctor, my baby is just two weeks old and always has this high fever.

A: A similar thing happened to my younger sister! A week and three days after she had her child; she called me to complain that the baby was running a fever. Now, I know my sister and how she likes to shroud her babies in layers and layers of warm clothes! You would almost think she lived somewhere in Antarctica as opposed to the hot tropics.

So, my first advice was for her to remove all the unnecessary 'chieftaincy' caps that I was sure she had wrapped the baby up in. It was a busy day, and I didn't call her back later that day. When I reached her the next day, she was very cheerful and said my advice worked like magic and once the baby was more lightly dressed, the fever disappeared! Magic, right? 😄 …Maybe not!

This is not a call to expose your baby to all manner of horrible weather, but really when it's warm, and you can clearly see the baby sweating, please do not make him or her wear a cardigan, jumper or sweater! I speak on behalf of all the poor, can't-talk neonates of Africa! 😄

Now, the above is a situation where there is really nothing wrong. However, fever in neonates can also be due to dehydration or infection.

More importantly, if your baby looks unwell use your thermometer to check the baby's temperature. The average body temperature is about 37° but if the baby's temperature is higher than this, please take your baby to see the paediatrician to make a proper diagnosis and start treatment. Ensure that you tepid sponge the baby all the way up till the doctor is seen to prevent convulsions due to fever, especially if there is a family history.

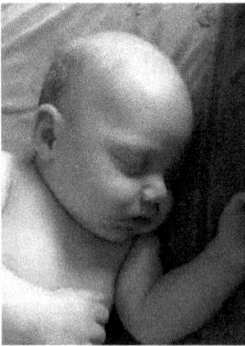

I AM EMBARRASSED BY THE BALD PATCHES ON MY SONS HEAD!!!

Q: Dr, please how do I treat ringworm on my son's head? We have treated it now for more than six months with various creams and shampoo still no result. Please, assist urgently as this is so embarrassing.

A: Fungal infection of the scalp, called Tinea Capitis, is often found in children and is commonly called ringworm too. If you're a parent and your child has had this, the embarrassment factor alone is significant enough to seek therapy. ☺

Parents try all sorts from the conventional to the not-so-conventional to take care of this. Anti-fungal creams, lotions and powders applied to the scalp don't quite work. Creative solutions like rubbing petrol on the scalp leaves you with a screaming child who still has holes and patches in his hair from the fungal infection. Where on earth, did that therapy come from? Petrol? Seriously!?! (Like my daughter would say ☺).

Tinea Capitis may involve all or some parts of the scalp. The involved areas may look bald and patchy with small, round spots from fallen hair, swollen and inflamed, etc. As is typical of fungal infections, they love moist and warm areas and will be encouraged to grow when one has a cut or bruise on the scalp, does not wash his or her hair regularly, sweats a lot and does not wash this off quickly and shares personal items of clothing like caps, hats, head scarves, towels, etc.

The infection can also be spread by coming in contact with ringworm on someone else's body or contacted from a pet.

Treatment is not achieved on the surface by using anti-fungal creams. This is achieved by taking anti-fungal drugs orally. This will usually be for a significant period of time- between six to eight weeks. Using anti-fungal shampoos may limit the spread of the infection but does not get rid of it. Again, even if signs of quick results are seen, this does not mean therapy should be stopped immediately. The drug should be taken for the full period prescribed by a doctor.

During the course of treatment, pillowcases, combs, towels and other items which are probably infected, should be disposed of, where possible. If not, they should be disinfected with bleach and washed in warm water. Subsequently, personal things should be kept personal and not shared with other people.

Personal hygiene is key, and children should be taught to take a bath, frequently too, especially after sweating. They should also stay away from stray dogs or those that have the infection (a bald patch on the dog's fur may be observed).

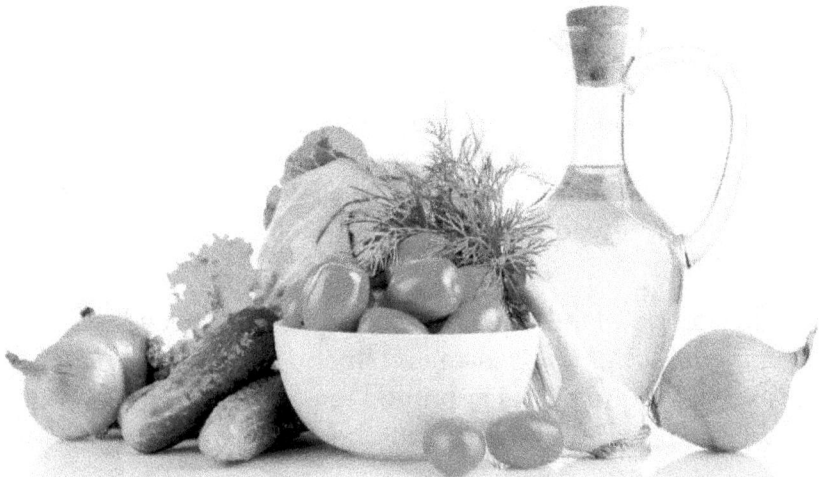

Diet Book

DR. NKECHI OLALERE

Verbatim Communications
Lagos, Nigeria

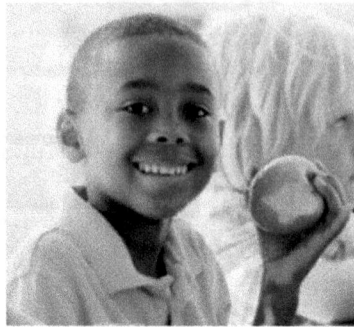

Introduction

DIET, EXERCISE AND SO MUCH MORE!

Over the years, I have given a 'gazillion' health talks. I've always said that I'm amazed by the fact that the questions never varied. Whether the health talk is given to top executives in a blue chip company or market women in a rural community, the questions are the same in content, even if not in grammar 😊

I was at a seminar some time late in 2013, and the title was 'what to eat and why.' We could barely get through the sessions. It was amazingly interactive, and people had a lot of questions to ask. The questions were sent to me in slips of papers, and I could not get around to answering all. So, I have decided to put the questions down in a book format hoping that it equips you with the information you'd asked for!

There are so many questions; this can only be Volume 1 at best!

Enjoy 😊

Part 1

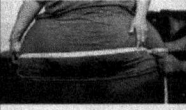

A SECOND ON THE LIPS,
A LIFETIME ON THE HIPS!

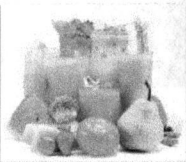

FRUITS

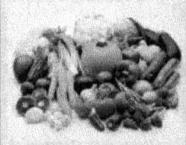

VEGETABLES

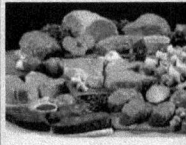

PROTEINS

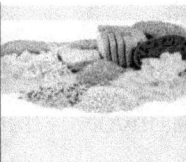

COMPLEX CARBOHYDRATES

A SECOND ON THE LiPS,
A LiFETiME ON THE HiPS!

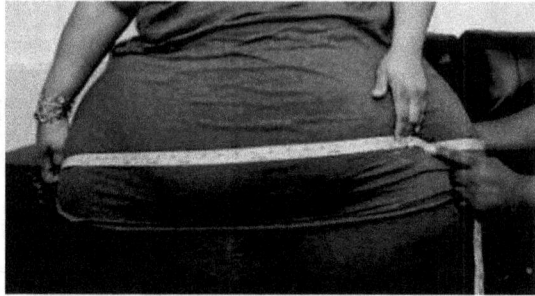

This piece is about healthy eating. The best of us would leave our good senses behind and 'pig-out' during celebrations and then suffer through the next couple of weeks trying to lose all that weight. Ever heard of, 'a second on the lips, a lifetime on the hips? Well, that certainly describes this.

There are all sorts of diets and eating regimens available, most of which impose the most amazing restrictions on our diets. But, these more often than not, result in yo-yo dieting...I'm on today and off tomorrow. However skewed toward a more realistic, conscious lifestyle modification that stands the test of time, involves things that are inculcated into everyday life decisions of what to eat and is more sustainable. What does this involve? Here goes:

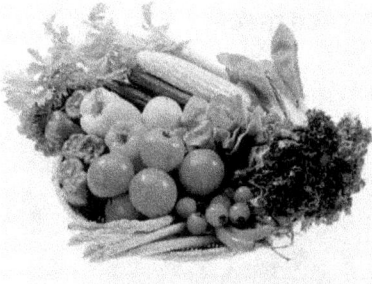

Eat more fruits and vegetables. Eating them in as close to their natural state as possible is, of course, more beneficial. We fall into the temptation of wanting to do the right thing as long as we're doing it on our terms; this would involve dousing these vegetables in oil and frying them. These vegetables are rich in Vitamin C, which is water soluble and so unnecessary cooking strips them of this nutrient. If we have got to cook them at all, add them at the final stage of cooking and cook for the barest minimum time; a minute or two.

Some of the veggies like carrots, lettuce or cabbage, are, of course, delicious eaten raw. These can be used in a salad with a dressing of balsamic vinegar or olive oil as opposed to all the fatty salad dressings out there. A recipe for salad dressing I learnt from the chef on my show, is yoghurt, honey and mustard dressing. Add a cup of yoghurt, a quarter cup of honey, 2 table spoons of mustard and 2 teaspoons of lemon juice. Whisk it all together and you've made for yourself a delicious dressing. The leaf of the garden egg, called akwukwo anara in Igbo (and efo Igbo in Yoruba, I believe?) is also delicious when eaten raw as a major part of the meal.

Talking about fruits and vegetables leads me to the question, 'how much of these can we realistically have in each meal?'

Well, the answer is probably not what you'd love to hear but happens to be true. For a standard dinner plate, half of it should be filled with fruits or vegetables, a quarter devoted to carbohydrates (carbs) and a quarter devoted to the protein component. The rule of thumb for the carbs is that it should not be more than the quantity in the cupped palm of one hand!

I hear your groans . 😊

For the petite people like me (this is more politically correct than saying, 'short' or one of the funniest ones I have heard, 'vertically challenged!'), this is a BIG problem! Close your eyes and visualise the tiny portions that can be accommodated in those tiny palms…sigh!

It is tough initially until your tummy adjusts to this portion…which is in little or no time. For the carbs, it would be great to focus on the complex carbs such as brown (Ofada) rice. This all boils down to portion control.

We talk about healthy oils like olive oils, canola oils but, even these contain pure fat. For example, there's about one-hundred and twenty

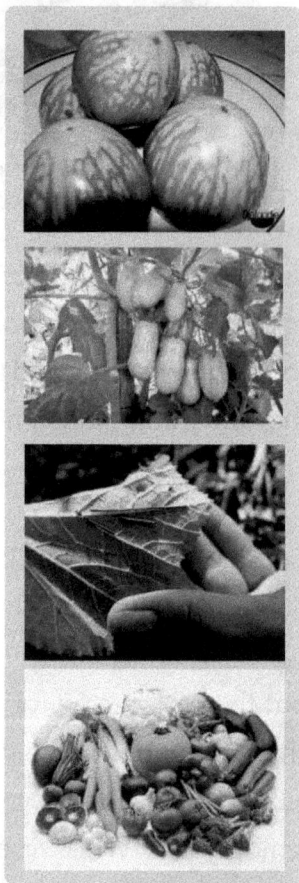

calories in each tablespoonful of olive oil, be it light or extra light. To put this in context, consider how much time it takes to burn off one hundred calories at the gym and the relative ease with which a tablespoon of oil goes onto our food.

Here's another example, if you take ten thousand steps each day through walking, jogging or running, you burn between three hundred to four hundred calories per day; less if you walk mainly flat surfaces! Yet, with one spoon of oil, more than a quarter of all that 'amazing hard work' has gone down the drain!

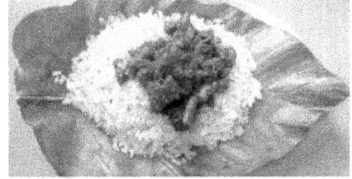

Imagine the number of activities involved in moving your feet ten thousand times in one day, compare it with the calories burnt and how much you gained by just adding a drop more oil. If this doesn't convince you to go easy on the oils, I don't know what else will! If you come from the Yoruba tribe (please be sure not to tell them I said this) 😊 then traditionally, cooking involves ladles and ladles of oils like palm oil which has a high content of saturated fats associated with high cholesterol levels. I remember the first time I was exposed to stew from the Yoruba race, it had so much oil that I couldn't see the tomatoes! Being a 'kobo-kobo' girl who was born into a tribe where we live on a diet of vegetables (in as raw a state as possible), that was a culture shock, and I never quite got used to it (please don't let my in-laws know that all that time I pretended to love those stews, I was just suffering through them) 😁

It was almost as great a culture shock as learning to kneel down to greet. I developed waist pain the first time we travelled to the village, what with all that kneeling which my okoro knees were not used to. 😄

The point is, use very little oil to cook…you don't need more than a spoon or two depending on what you're cooking. I hear you groaning and wondering how this will taste, but you could try and re-train your taste buds. Let them get used to less oil and even less salt.

Talking about salt, are you one of those who routinely use the salt-shaker in their food even before they taste it? Well, that is a habit that's got to be tossed away. Salt has been implicated in different studies as a major cause of hypertension. The rule of thumb is, 'if you can taste it, it's probably too much!'.

This is not a discourse aimed at forcing you into an existence where you are 'simply living' and not enjoying your life through tasty meals…after all, a couple of my friends tell me, 'na something go kill person.' So we live in the moment, enjoy it and go out with a bang!

Well, that's certainly an option.   I hear you thinking (don't ask me how I hear people think. I've got psychic powers like that!) "The food that I get to eat using these suggestions is definitely going to be bland!" Nope, they don't have to be. Use spices to add that extra special zing to your food. Thyme, curry and garlic are some good examples of heart-friendly spices to use in food and give it a little 'something extra.'

Endeavour not to skip meals because when you do, you compensate for this later and binge. So for breakfast eat like a king (buttressing the importance of breakfast), for lunch, eat like a prince and for dinner, eat like a pauper!

Breakfast could be a nourishing bowl of oatmeal. For those of you who hate it, like my children, cinnamon, which has amazing health benefits including lowering cholesterol makes it tastier. You could also cut up apples and bananas into it and add some raisins/dried fruits for an extra sugar kick. Lunch could be wheat meal with vegetable soup and fish while dinner could be something light like moi-moi. Remember to follow the cooking instructions and serving portions…a handful. An acceptable way of circumventing this or increasing the portion available is to grow taller and of course increase hand span. He he he! Let's see you try. 😁

FRUiTS

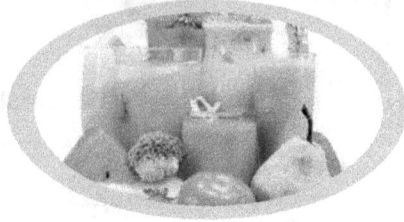

Q: How much fruit should I eat in a day and which fruits are the best to eat?

A: Fruits are part of a healthy diet, and everyone should have at least five servings in a day. However, fruits are also high in sugars such as fructose and this has been linked to weight gain and chronic diseases like Diabetes Mellitus. Ordinarily, this fructose shouldn't be a problem, but the thing is with our love for 'sugar rush' people are getting even more sugar from other sources apart from fruits. Cumulatively, this sugar load becomes a problem.

According to studies carried out on these nutritional items, it has been discovered that some fruits have more sugar content than others. The following have been arranged in increasing order of their sugar contents: Blackberries,

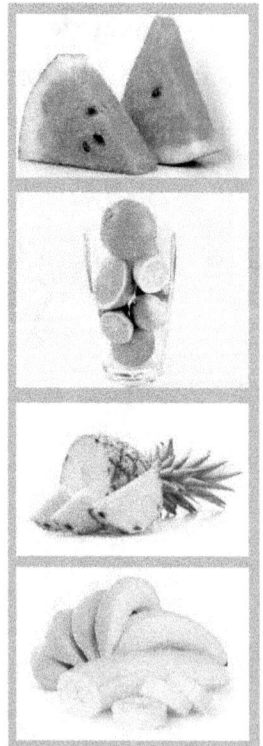

strawberries, apples, pineapples, oranges, bananas and grapes. This means that blackberries have less fructose than strawberries and strawberries have less than apples etc.

Super-fruits are given their unique name because they are full of vitamins, minerals, anti-oxidants and fibre which works together to keep you healthy and even prevent diseases. Some of them are apples, bananas, blackberries, blueberries, cherries, oranges, lemon, lime, grapefruit, watermelon, pineapples, pawpaw, etc.

Q: Are supplements good alternatives to fruits and vegetables?

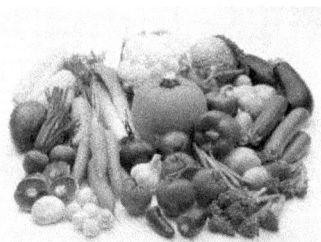

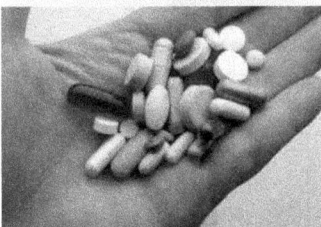

A: Nothing beats a healthy diet filled with fruits and vegetables to keep you healthy and equipped to fight all manner of diseases. Supplements, as the name implies are meant to plug in the tiny holes that may not be completely filled by your diet. For instance, if your diet regularly misses out on dairy products despite the recommendation of at least three servings per day, you probably need calcium and Vitamin D supplements.

If, however, you're a junk food lover, there's no magic pill that can take care of your problem. What you need is a menu make-over focusing on portion control and right-plating with the different food groups. Remember that to plate right, half your plate should be filled with fruits and vegetables, a quarter with proteins and the last quarter with complex carbohydrates.

Q: Does this diet of fruits, vegetables and whole grains apply to children? I feel that, because they are growing, they need sugar and the like.

A: You are certainly right. They need sugar to fuel all that activity that makes parents continually yell, 'what's going on there?' 😊 But, it's probably not the type of sugar that you know, i.e. refined sugar from baked goods, soft drinks, etc.

All the food we eat eventually gets converted to sugar in the body and the sugar from refined products causes sugar spikes and lows such that the people who eat them, get hungry very quickly after they felt full, so limit the sugar from this source. However, sugar from other sources like complex carbs are released slowly causing a feeling of fullness for longer.

As parents or caregivers, we have to model the right food behaviour for our children. We can't tell them to take fruits and then turn around to take soda. In the same vein, we can't eat junk and expect them to grow up and have healthy food habits. Another thing we do, which may promote the wrong image of food in children, is that we oftentimes give them sweets or candy as a reward for good behaviour. Therefore, it's only natural for them to now desire this.

Wondering what they should eat? Pretty much the same diet requirements as you but with varying calorie needs at different ages.

Serve a variety of fruits and vegetables, especially those in season. They are cheap and readily available. And remember that fruit juices are not as good as fresh fruits themselves because they are loaded with sugar and even if you don't see sugar on the label, the 'concentrate' you do see is loaded with it! The exception to this would be 100% fruit juice.

Seafood, beans, eggs and unsalted nuts are good protein sources. Dairy is also a good source of protein. Once a child is about two years old, please switch to skimmed or one to two percent milk. Cheese, yoghurt and soy drinks are also great dairy options.

Whole grains are also found in brown/local rice, oats, whole wheat bread and popcorn (yep, popcorn 😊) provide complex carbs and fibre for that feeling of fullness and of course great bowel movement with no constipation. But be sure not to douse them with sugar or salt'. You can grill some chicken or stir fry some minced chicken or beef with onions and some spices and then use this to make a sandwich using whole grain bread.

Keep healthy snacks around the house like nuts, fruits and vegetables that can be dipped in sauces, yoghurt or other dips.

VEGETABLES

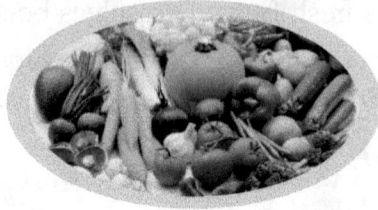

Q: I always have problems with eating vegetables. Whenever I eat it, it makes me stool. Why?

A: Well, apart from the anti-oxidants that are available in fruits and vegetables, one of the main functions of vegetables is also to provide dietary fibre (roughage) which add bulk to your stool and ensures that you have regular bowel movement; thus preventing constipation. So, it should make you stool! 😁

This fibre is not digested by your body and so passes by, almost unchanged which is why it promotes a feeling of fullness without the accompanying calories.

Apart from normalizing your bowel movement, it also helps lower cholesterol level and can aid you in achieving a healthy weight because you need more chewing time for this - so, your brain has time to receive the message that your tummy is full - and because they are bulky, you feel full.

Foods rich in fibre include beans, peas, apples, carrots, oats, citrus fruits, green leafy veggies etc. When cooking foods like beans or green leafy vegetables, be sure not to smother them in oil. It defeats the whole essence of healthy eating, doesn't it?

PROTEINS

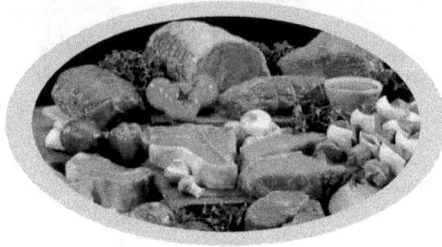

Q: You didn't talk about plant protein.

A: Plant proteins, except soya beans, do not have all the essential amino acids. They are called complementary vegetable proteins. Complementary proteins are proteins that lack one or more essential amino acids (building blocks of proteins) required to keep the body functioning properly. These include most proteins of plant origin except soya beans. When incomplete proteins are paired together, they produce complete proteins.

Here are complementary protein groups with examples;

- Seeds–pumpkin (Egusi) seeds, sunflower seeds, sesame seeds

- Grains – oats, wheat, rice (brown/local), barley, corn bread, pasta (like whole wheat macaroni/spaghetti), dumplings, biscuits.

- Nuts–walnuts (Asala, Awusa), cashews, almonds, pistachios

- Legumes – soy products, beans, peas, peanuts.

What are the best combinations?

Grains and legumes e.g. Rice and beans, corn and beans, peanut butter (groundnut paste) on wheat bread or biscuits, oats with some peanuts thrown in (I like that!).

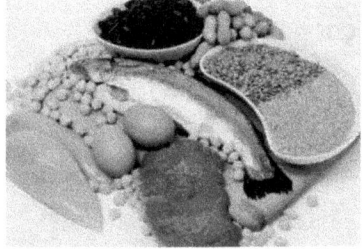

These are great combinations.
Legumes and seeds e.g. peanuts and pumpkin seeds as a snack is another great combination.

Grains and seeds e.g. wheat meal or oatmeal paste with Egusi soup is a good combination.

Other protein sources are:

Dairy: Low fat (e.g. Greek) yoghurt, low fat or skimmed milk, cheese. Some dairy and vegetable protein sources also make complete proteins. E.g. dairy and grains (cheese on wheat bread or biscuit is a great combination)

Eggs: Make sure the egg is properly boiled to prevent Salmonella infection Canned tuna. So, there you go.

Q: How many eggs should I eat in a day and are eggs healthy to eat?

A: Over the years, we have heard many things about eggs...all of them bad! 👀 And really, no one is to blame for this because it was found that egg yolks contain a lot of cholesterol; as a result nobody wanted any part of it.

However, recent studies have suggested that the amount of cholesterol in eggs plays a smaller role in increasing our total blood cholesterol than saturated fats present in cookies, pastries, cakes, etc. In essence, this means that saturated fats in our cookies et al. stand a better chance of increasing blood cholesterol than eggs. That is certainly cheery news.

Nevertheless, I would say, that just like for seafood, which also has a high amount of cholesterol, if you have high cholesterol levels, it may be wise to limit your egg intake to occasional treats or speak with your doctor before embarking on a binge.

Generally, one egg per day should be fine for other people.

Eggs are chock full of proteins, vitamins and minerals and have only eighty-five calories in one; thus, they are great breakfast options for people watching their weight as they feel full for a longer period of time. However, it may be a wise idea to switch this up on different days of the week with oats or other cereals for breakfast to increase our intake of fibre that helps reduce blood cholesterol. Another option is a boiled egg on a piece of whole wheat toast.

Ensure that your eggs are well cooked. In fact, pregnant women, children, old people and generally, people who are unwell should only eat eggs whose yolk and egg whites have been boiled till its solid

Also, store the eggs in their boxes in the fridge and try to finish egg dishes as soon as possible.

Q: What about hides and skin (Ponmo)? Are they nutritious and is it healthier to eat Ponmo instead of red meat?

A: I will start by saying that I know that we all love our ponmo and the delicious, succulent texture it has in our mouth. When it has been well boiled and seasoned, it literally melts in your mouth! There's just nothing like it! For all the non-Africans or perhaps, non-West Africans reading this, you will be absolutely amazed to imagine that I am describing the skin or hide of cows! Yep! That was not an error. And we love this delicacy. 😄

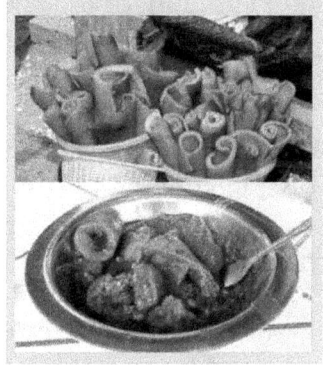

Most unfortunately, this well-loved delicacy is devoid of any nutritional value. In fact, if you do a quick web search, the first quick information you would get about cow skin is how to harness this to make shoes, belts and other leather goods.

Hence, if the options were ponmo or red meat, the 'obvious' answer would be red meat (with all the fat trimmed out). Or better still, chicken (breast is a better option than the darker meat), fish etc.

Now, I know that beyond the fact that we have elevated ponmo to an 'art-form' delicacy, the reason a lot of people eat it is because it's cheap and was thought to be an alternative source of protein. So, where do we go from here for cheap protein sources? I'll help you solve this problem:

Try complementary vegetable proteins as described in the previous section.

Q: Are snails, crabs and prawns healthy to eat?

A: Seafood is generally safe because it contains a good amount of protein and Omega 3 fatty acids which are very healthy. They are also low in calories and rich in a lot of minerals like Zinc, Selenium and vitamins such as B12. Nonetheless, snails, crabs, prawns and shrimps are also pretty high in cholesterol and so should be taken as an occasional treat by people who have high cholesterol.

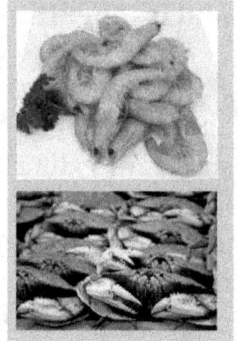

Other issues to note include:

- ⊙ Shrimps, prawns and crabs are best taken fresh rather than frozen. When frozen, they have a whole lot more sodium…probably from the salt used as a preservative, and this could increase blood pressure.

- ⊙ Avoid raw, under-cooked or uncooked seafood and shellfish especially when pregnant. Make sure prawns and shrimps are a milk white colour when cooked.

- ⊙ Generally, when pregnant, the main concern is the amount of mercury in the fish or seafood. Large mackerel, Swordfish, Tilefish and Shark contain a large amount of Mercury that could cause defects in the baby's developing nervous system.

As for all you sushi lovers, give the Japanese treat a rest when pregnant especially if it is made with any of the fishes listed above.

COMPLEX CARBOHYDRATES

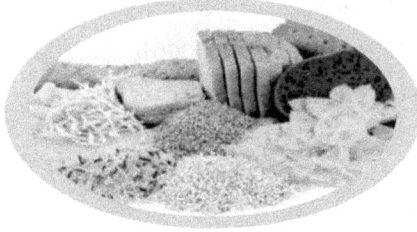

Q: When you eat only eba, beans, rice and bread, is it dangerous?

A: I came across a report from a Harvard review, and it gives eight principles to low glycemic eating. If you reduce your portion sizes and are exercising and generally doing the right things, you may still be adding weight or not losing weight if you're eating a lot of food with high glycemic index.

Glycemic index, by the way, is a measure that ranks foods that contain carbohydrates on a scale of 0 to 100. The higher the number, the faster the food, is digested, causing fluctuations in the blood sugar level and the lower the number, the slower the food is digested causing fewer fluctuations in the blood sugar level. So the focus should be on foods with low glycemic index.

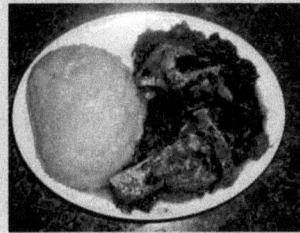

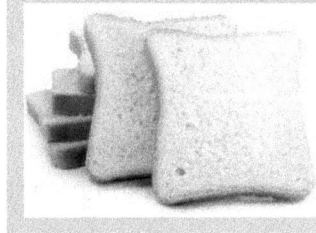

These are the principles of low glycemic eating:

- ⊙ Eat a lot of beans, non-starchy veggies like garlic, onions, leeks, chives, cabbage, broccoli, lettuce, tomatoes or peppers and fruits such as apples, berries, peaches and pears.

- ⊙ Chew a lot of grains in their natural state like natural granola, brown or local rice and muesli cereal.

- ⊙ Reduce your intake of concentrated sweets like fruit juices (no more than half a cup daily, if you must) and other sugar-loaded or sweetened drinks.

- ⊙ Load up on healthy proteins like fish, skinless chicken and beans…again.

- ⊙ Cut down on your intake of refined grain products like white bread and polished rice.

- ⊙ Minimize your daily consumption of bad fats by avoiding fast-foods and limiting your intake of animal products. Focus on healthy oils like Olive oil and nuts like almonds. However, even these should be taken in moderation as even healthy oils are full of calories! It appears you just can't win!

- ⊙ Be sure to take your breakfast and eat three meals with a snack or two (healthy options, of course).

- ⊙ Finally, remember to eat slowly to give enough time for your stomach to tell your brain that you're full…and then stop!

Part 2

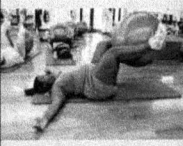 DIET

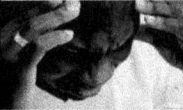 EXERCISE

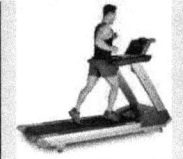 STRESS

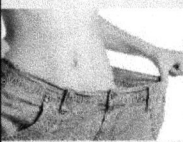 JOHNNY WALKER

WEIGHT LOSS
(FACTS AND FICTIONS)

DIET

This is very critical in terms of what you eat, how you eat it and how much of it is eaten. A meal filled with junk food i.e. meat pies and doughnuts, is unhealthy on a lot of fronts. It contains empty calories you don't need and makes you demand even more food in a short while. They also cause your blood sugar to yo-yo - jump up and down - in a way that doesn't help blood sugar control.

A diet that is also full of white carbs like white bread and polished rice is also not ideal for the same reason. So what should we eat? A balanced diet...one that contains all food groups in sufficient amounts for the body to use them efficiently.

Over time, I have had cause to describe the ideal plate of food and this is the basic structure: Half the plate should be filled with vegetables, a quarter with complex carbohydrates like beans, local rice (Ofada, Abakaliki, brown or wild rice), sweet potatoes or oatmeal and the last quarter with protein which could be fish, chicken or other types of healthy meat.

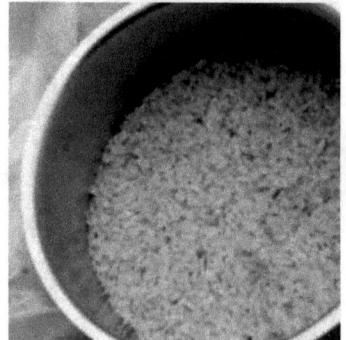

For the record, not all carbs are created equal. Complex carbs are superior because they supply energy and fibre and some also supply minerals and vitamins. In the light of this, note that they are necessary to provide the energy needed for our daily activities. So, do not 'demonise' them.

Do not forget portion control. Reduce the plate size you usually use, if you need to lose weight as this automatically reduces the quantity of food you can eat.

Remember also to make a conscious effort to chew your food properly and take your time. Don't wolf it down…or inhale it.

Chew intentionally so as to give your brain sufficient time to process the signal which says that your stomach is full. Have you observed that when you rush your food, you move from being very hungry to being completely stuffed! There's no in-between, where you realize that you're full before you get to the stuffed part. That's because your brain didn't have enough time to process that info before you became 'over-full'.

Note that, even if a meal is considered healthy, it doesn't mean you should eat as much of it as you want. For instance, beans are healthy on so many levels but it is also high in calories and so you still need to stick to the portion described.

Moderation in everything!

THE TRiO OF DiET, EXERCiSE AND STRESS

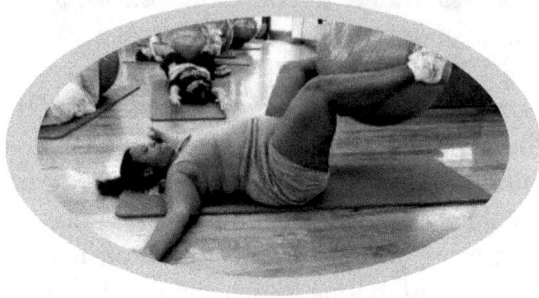

Exercise is critical because it makes your heart strong, improves your body's ability to break down food, resist diseases and generally provides a feel-good attitude. It also helps you lose weight.

Mathematically, exercise helps to burn what you have eaten such that, if you do enough and watch your portions, at the end of the day, there will be a good balance between what you have burnt and what you have taken in. If you have not been engaged in any exercise for a long time, please see your doctor before you start any vigorous regimen. A minimum of 150 minutes of exercise per week is essential for good health. Try to get this exercise anyway you can by walking, dancing, skipping, arm wrestling or even pillow fights. All the activities count and help you keep you fit, trim and healthy. If you use the gym, that's great. You can get an instructor to put you on a regimen that involves aerobics, strength training (training with weights) and then focus on troublesome spots like your tummy (in that order) or suggest useful regimens that are helpful.

Finally, I will talk about stress because quite a number of us are stressed out and as we approach festive periods like the end of the year with all the activities involved, we get even more stressed out.

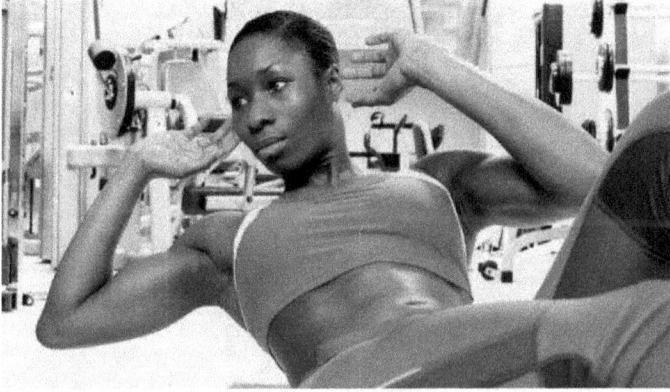

STRESS

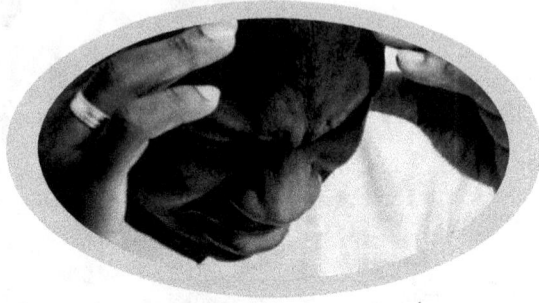

This thing called stress!

I see it in my face in the mornings when I wake up. I see it in my neighbours' faces; in traffic…even my children are not immune to it! Why are we all stressed? Where are we all rushing to? What's to win in this rat race? So many questions…but there are no quick answers.

In that tiny corner of my mind, a little voice says, 'But the holy book says that with a little more sleep comes poverty,' so I have got to be busy doing something at all times. But…wait a moment! Am I doing productive stuff? Am I actually staving off poverty with this activity that doesn't quite appear to be leading me anywhere I want to go? Am I sweating the small stuff? Getting worked up over issues I have no control over? Now, I have managed to ask even more questions!

For the answers…I wish I could say I knew them all. But I do know that we can't cope when we have bitten off more than we can chew. I will use myself as an example. Busy career woman (kinda sounds cool to describe myself that way) 😊 with children and multiple interests in wellness, training and facilitation which keep me pretty busy twenty-four hours of every day.

I start each day with a long list of things that I have to accomplish. Some days, I am lucky, and I get through them all. Some other days...okay, let's be truthful here...most days, I don't get to finish that list. But I have learnt to look at my cup as half full as opposed to half empty. At the end of the day, I am thankful to God for how far I have gone, and I keep the undone ones in the cooler and start the next day in as sequential an order as I can manage.

In the office, I try to focus on the major issues and leave the rest of the team to handle the clutter (first lesson in how not to micro-manage!). And at home...you will probably wonder at my craziness when you hear my solution to house helps that drive you mad!

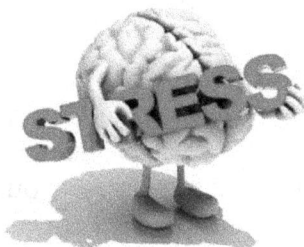

First, get your children involved in the household chores and cooking...yes, you heard me right: the cooking! I think, from my experience, that this makes the housekeeper understand that you do have an option in terms of keeping or not keeping them. Then, when we are off to work and school, I lock up the house, and she is free to spend her day as she likes...sleeping or anything that takes her fancy. This way when I get back I am not upset about how dirty or not clean everywhere looks. The work can start when I get back or over the weekend. Now I know that for those of you who have younger children, this may not work because you do need someone to be there in the house twenty-four hours a day, seven days a week and I get that. So work out a system that works for you and remember that the sooner you can get your children to start cleaning up after themselves, the better. The main focus should be on getting you less aggravated and more relaxed.

Eat healthy, walk about ten thousand steps a day (did I hear you say, how? I'll tell you in another book), catch as much sleep as you can: in the car (when you are not driving, of course), to work as well as to and from appointments and try to get to bed early. Limit the distractions in your room when it is bedtime (TV et al.) and eat light in the evenings.

Most importantly, don't sweat the small stuff...the report was not done the right way, just show them how; the place was not properly cleaned, tell them to repeat it; the nanny didn't wash the clothes well, save up for and get a washing machine; someone cuts into your lane in traffic...resist the urge to give him some home truths! Who knows....maybe with these we can actually win the rat race!

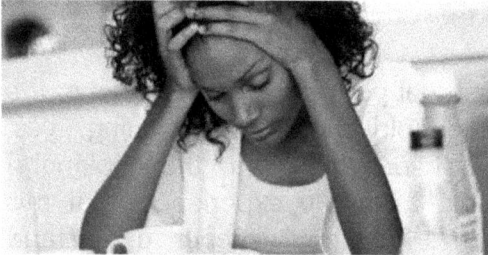

Stress causes the release of a hormone called Cortisol which, amongst other things, causes fat to be deposited around our tummy. The bad thing about tummy-fat is that it is not on the outside. It is actually on the inside, around the organs. So, no amount of sit-ups can touch this fat...it can help tighten abdominal muscles (especially for those who just gave birth) but it won't get to the fat around organs (visceral fat).

This fat is associated with disease conditions like Diabetes Mellitus. So, reduce your stress consciously by figuring out how to better cope with your sources of stress or even eliminating the stressors that you have control over. It's your life after all.

Johnny Walker!

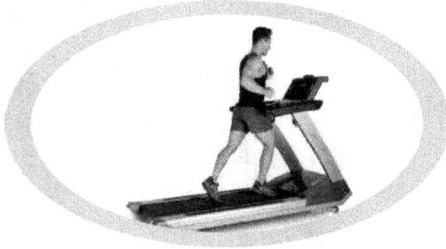

Okay! This is certainly not what you thought when you saw the subject; I assure you! But, hey…don't leave…at least not just yet. Not until you have read what I have got to say!

Yes, this is not a post extolling the virtue of this prime drink neither is this meant to disrespect it. Nope! This is in honour of the time worn, aged, good old fashioned ancient means of transportation called 'Walking'!

Don't roll your eyes!

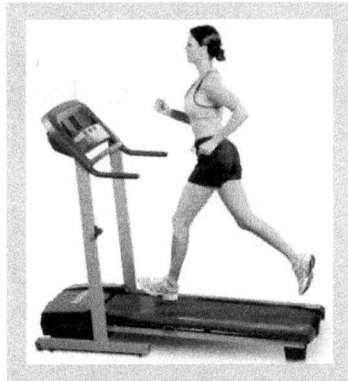

Okay, if I ask, how many times you've gone to the gym in the past one year? What would be the answer? If I asked, how many times you've been able to clock up to 150 minutes of exercise in a week? What if I asked, what your daily routine is? Would it sound like…from the house, to the car, to the office, back to the car, off to meetings, back to the car and off to the house? Does this sound like you? Well, you are not alone! It took the magical object called a pedometer to bring to my attention how little I was moving around when I stopped going to the gym due to some 'household operational challenges' (code for 'my nanny up and left without notice! 😌). The first day I used it; I racked up all of four hundred and thirty-two steps!!! Did you get that? In all of the twenty-four hours; I moved my feet one way or the other a total of four hundred and thirty-two times! That is pathetic! And really scary given that a **sedentary lifestyle** (one in which there is little **physical activity**), can increase our risks of hypertension, obesity, cancers, diabetes, etc.

Even our children are not left out! I usually park a little distance away from the church on **Sundays**, just so that immediately after the service, we can make a quick escape without having to wait for people to move their cars. But my children hate the very idea of that short walk to where the car is parked, and they will use any opportunity to whine about it!

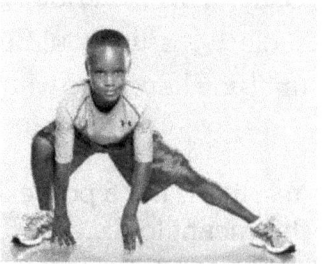

Okay, what's the answer to this? Get physical! Go out and play football, table tennis, **basketball, lawn tennis** with your spouse, the children and friends. This ensures you're getting the required exercise and also bonding with your family.

Visit the gym and do weight trainings or aerobics. Did I hear you say 'oh, but I work so hard and I can hardly find time to sleep, how much more exercise?' Then find other ways of doing this. Instead of calling the Accounts Department to find out the status of that invoice, walk across there, instead of using the elevators, use the stairs. Instead of being driven all the way to your front door, stop at your gate and walk the rest of the way inside and instead of calling the nanny to get you water, go get it yourself. In all of this, the goal is to rack up thirty minutes of exercise at least five days a week and if you are using a pedometer, at least ten thousand steps per day!

Okay! I heard all the screams of ten thousand? Was that a mistake? Did you mean to say one thousand? Nope! I meant and still mean ten thousand. Now, this is the optimal. However, if you are starting out from the very depths where I started, then aim to increase your steps by at least five hundred per week until you get to the Promised Land. You'll be amazed at the fun activities that can rack up steps quickly.

If you love your Owambes, enjoy and be sure to dance! Not the stationary 'hips down, backside swaying kinda dance...nope! More like the Nkpokiti, atiolgwu or salsa dance steps (hmmm! writing these three dance steps together raises interesting imagery right here! Beyonce, eat your heart out!). You've got to get some motion in there! You know all those stuff your children want you to do...like carry them around, swing them around or just chase after them? They all count!

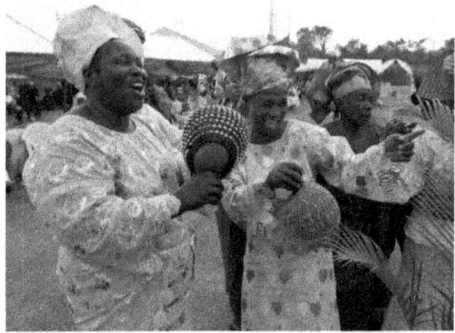

Every little step counts towards making you **healthier** and happier! Celebrate every milestone with five thousand being the first major one. This takes you firmly out of a sedentary lifestyle group and on your way to wellness!

Numerically, 5,000-7,499 steps per day is termed "low active." 7,500-9,999 is considered "somewhat active" and ten thousand steps per day indicate the point at which an individual is classified as "active". People who take more than twelve thousand five hundred steps per day are classified as "highly active".

So start small, keep at it, get those joints to stop creaking and keep those terrible diseases at bay! Keep walking people!

Weight loss (facts and fiction)

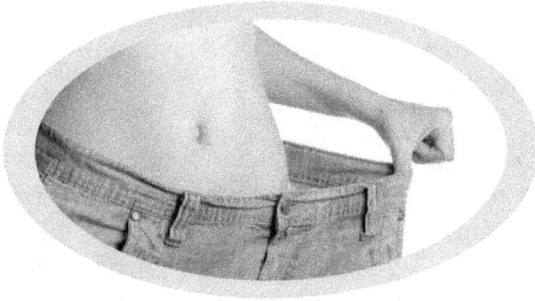

There is so much to talk about weight loss, and I will also try to weigh in on some facts and fiction too.

I have a lot of people who write in and tell me that they don't know why they add weight because they hardly eat! Now, I have never seen anyone who stays off food and actually gains weight. That would be an interesting study! For this group, the main problem is what they actually eat, whenever they eat.

Tips To Lose Weight

1. Keep a Food Journal
2. Drink 6 Cups of Water A Day
3. Eat More Greens
4. Cook With Fat Free Broth
5. Eat Whole Grains
6. Measure Everything
7. Use Skim Milk
8. Take Your Time Eating
9. Use Smaller Plates
10. Exercise
11. Eat More Seafood
12. Use Meat as a Condiment
13. Eat More Fiber
14. Eat More Vegetarian Meals
15. Eat Healthy Snacks

Other times, people tell me, the only thing I've eaten all day is biscuits and a bottle of soft drink. However, the thing about biscuits and soft drinks is that they contain empty calories which give you a quick feeling of fullness, rapidly followed by more hunger pangs…and then you find yourself reaching for more biscuits. If, however, you were to eat a complex carbohydrate or even fruits, they keep you feeling fuller for longer, and you avoid the temptation to eat more.

Some people also write in to ask me about slimming pills or green tea or any of those wonder drugs that make you shed weight in 'seconds' and instruct you never to eat of specific classes of foods. Let's use green tea as an example. Green tea is great, and studies have shown that it speeds up metabolism, therefore; it helps you break down all the food you swallowed, faster.

On the other hand, weight gain is a function of what you've taken in and what you've taken out. If you take in three thousand calories and you're able to burn only five hundred calories, then clearly, there is some excess that will get converted to fat and other components. Remember that some of our 'snacks' such as burgers pack as much as five hundred to six hundred calories in one serving….and that's just one meal (or maybe even one snack) with three more meals and perhaps another snack before the day draws to a close. So, if you are loading your system with more food than you need, then even the purest of green tea is going to have a hard time keeping up with your metabolism…there is just too much work to do with all that food! 😃

Remember that generally, women are entitled to two thousand calories intake in a day and men are entitled to two thousand five hundred.

Some wonder if they can lose weight without exercise. They can…if they watch their dietary portions. However, exercise is useful for more than just weight loss. Exercise makes your heart strong and reduces the risk of other ailments.

Another popular question I am asked on a regular basis is; "I eat only once a day, how can I possibly add weight with that?"

If you eat once a day, chances are you snack on other things during the day that you do not consider as food…it could very well be cookies, etc. But even if you don't snack on anything, chances are that when you eat once, you binge and essentially makeup for all the meals that you didn't eat during the day....and so we are back to square one. 😊

Remember that you are actually allowed up to five small meals in a day; three main meals and two snacks. These are some points to ponder as we go about our business and our parties.

Q: How many meals should I eat in a day?

A: The jury is really still out on this one. One school of thought insists that small mini-meals every two to three hours is great and improves metabolism. The other school of thought claims that there is no significant finding that confirms that this is any better than the regular three square meals we have been used to.

Well, worldwide, we are all agreed on the fact that more proteins, fruits, veggies and complex carbs are the way to go. If you add portion control to the mix ensuring that you have the right amount of food with fruits and veggies making up half of the plate; complex carbs taking up, a quarter of the plate and proteins in the last part of the plate, then you should be good. At this point, it won't really matter whether you're doing six mini-meals or three main meals all day...you will still be able to keep the weight off (with some exercise in the mix too) and really just be healthy.

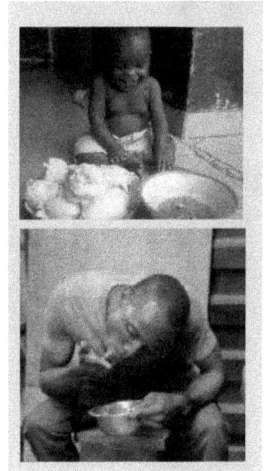

Q: I don't take alcohol. Both my parents have big tummies. I am of average build, but my tummy gives me concern. What do I do to keep my tummy down?

A: It's great that you are concerned about this, especially knowing that there is a family history, because genetics can be a factor in the issue of belly fat, also known as central obesity. However, other major factors are really what we eat, how much of it we eat and how much exercise we get. If you ensure that your plate always has all food groups in it, you'll be fine.

Give more attention to controlling the portion of food you ingest. The first practical step in doing this is to reduce the size of the plate that you ordinarily eat with. After which you need to ensure that half of this plate is filled with vegetables, a quarter of it with protein and the last quarter with the carbs.

For carbohydrates, focus on the complex carbohydrates like brown rice, local rice (Abakaliki or Ofada rice), sweet potatoes, oatmeal, whole wheat bread or millet. For instance, you can have half a plate filled with vegetables (remember to go extra easy on the oil during preparation), quarter of the plate filled with whole wheat meal and then your protein of choice, preferably fish or poultry. It is important to have more of the vegetables because these fill you up, absorb loads of fluid and keep you feeling fuller for longer!

You are also allowed 2-3 snacks daily but it's healthy ones like nuts and fruits that should be taken. And then exercise. I am always asked if people can lose weight without exercise and the answer is yes. I mean, if you went on a starvation diet, you would lose weight, right? 😁

But it's not sustainable.

First it's really water weight you are getting rid of, and you are not really imbibing the principles of a healthy lifestyle that will help you not only lose weight, but keep it off. Current recommendation is for

150 minutes of exercise weekly. This should be broken down into thirty minutes for five days of the week or one hour for three days. Space these minutes out and ensure that you don't try to get all of it done in two days like some weekend warriors I know. 😀 Seriously though, the heart may not be able to withstand that much pressure all at once having been sedentary too long. So, please be guided! 😜

Ageing also plays a role. However, if you start early enough in life to eat right, it may not be too much of a problem later. Visceral fat, the type involved in central obesity may not be helped much by abdominal exercises, crunches et al. This is why the right lifestyle is critical. Remember that central obesity pre-disposes one to heart diseases, Type 2 Diabetes Mellitus and so on. I'm sure you don't want to be here if you can do something about it!

Part 3

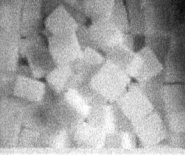 SUGAR RUSH

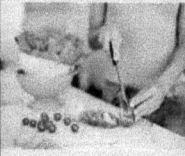 PREPARING AND COOKING YOUR VEGGIES

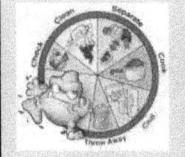 PREVENTION OF CROSS-CONTAMINATION OF FOOD

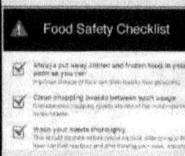 DAILY HEALTH TIPS: FOOD HYGIENE

SUGAR RUSH!

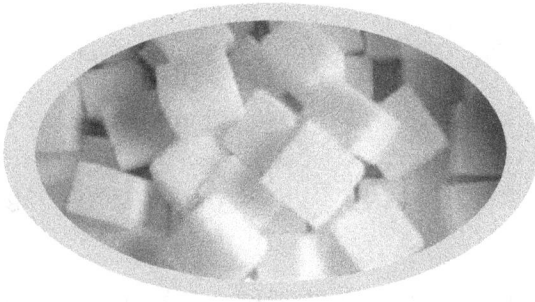

Q: Is the popular belief that when I take a lot of sugary things I can become diabetic true?

A: Well, it is not a lie. But it's not just the sugary nature of the food that's a problem. These foods are processed, depriving the body of the real nutrients they require. They are empty calories and so eating them floods the blood stream with sugar which quickly dissipates leaving the person hungry again and desiring yet another sugar fix!

Other starchy foods are also culprit. Eating too much leads to over flooding of the blood stream with simple sugars which may overwhelm the pancreas that produce insulin. Complex carbs, on the other hand, cause a more gradual increase in blood sugar, which is better for you.

In the past, Diabetes Mellitus (DM) was a disease associated with old age. For young people, this wasn't really an issue and it wasn't very common to see children with insulin injections setting up shots. But it's not such a rarity anymore.

A couple of weeks ago, in church, the Pastor shared a story of a child brought into the hospital who did not have any obvious signs of illness but on investigation, it was realised that she was diabetic. The blood glucose level was so high she had to be kept in the hospital for treatment. The poor girl was confused…'why am I being kept in the hospital when I am not even ill?' - at least she didn't feel ill. But for her parents, things had changed…very radically! This beautiful child they have was to be consigned to a life of pills and injections.

Now, pills and injections are a good thing if they preserve life and indeed improve or at least do not negatively alter the quality of life of the person taking them. But perhaps there's something we can do to stop the relentless march of this scourge?

To put things in context, let's discuss briefly what Diabetes Mellitus (DM)is. Usually, the food we eat is converted to simple sugars inside our bodies after which an organ of the body; the pancreas, secretes insulin that moves these sugars into the cells. In DM, this doesn't happen as the body does not respond to the stimulus of glucose in the blood by releasing insulin or is unable to produce insulin.

There are two types of DM: Type 1 and Type 2. In Type 1; which usually occurs in children, the insulin secreting cells are destroyed, so there is no insulin to send the glucose into the cells. In the latter, the cells of the body that produce insulin are no longer able to do so when there is a load of sugar in the blood. They become insensitive to the sugar stimulus.

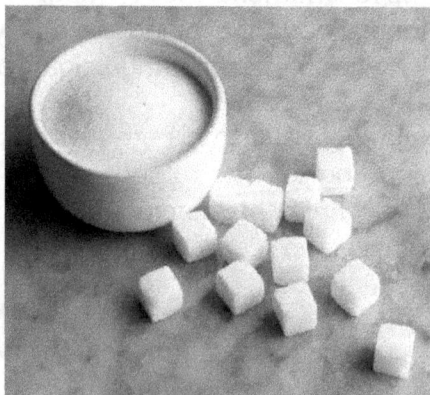

Wondering what to do to prevent Diabetes Mellitus in our childrenand ourselves…especially for those who are already pre-diabetic (people with higher than normal glucose levels but not high enough to be called diabetic) or have a family history of DM; bearing in mind that this will mostly work for Type 1 DM? Two words of advice: stay active and stay lean.

Staying active involves engaging in some physical activity every day. Most of us live sedentary lifestyles now and hardly involve ourselves in activities or encourage our children to. All those video and computer games we buy for our children have taken over their lives...well, sort of. They plop down in front of them merrily chasing the characters along their way and watching all manner of shows: learning things we want them to (maybe) and the ones we are shocked actually gets shown on TV!

Staying lean involves eating healthy by making sure that we practise portion control. Half our plates should be filled with veggies, a quarter with protein and a quarter with complex carbs (yam, potatoes, beans, etc.). Discover the different veggies available in the market or grocery shop and find a way of incorporating these into your meal plan.

Other healthy measures you can take are: quit smoking, reduce alcohol intake and reduce the consumption of processed foods.

So next time you feel the need for a sugar fix remember the fact that this second of pleasure may end with a lifetime of pain.

Q: Sugar cane or sweet soft drinks. How should I take them in a week?

A: Food is very important to life and health. Some foods are particularly important as they help build our immunity against certain diseases. In the same vein, research has shown that some foods when eaten regularly set us up for disease conditions like Diabetes Mellitus, hypertension and even cancers. Listed are some of such foods, and they should rarely be eaten.

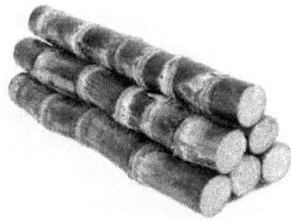

⊙ Added sugar from all sources- white sugar, brown sugar, soft

- drinks and other artificially sweetened products - make your blood sugar rise and fall erratically. And they contain empty calories that do not help you at all.

- Baked goodies like cakes, doughnuts and pies contain a lot of unhealthy fats, processed carbs and of course, added sugar.

- Processed meats like bacon, sausages and ham are certainly not as healthy as white meat such as skinless chicken. Fish is also a good alternative.

- Dairy foods like full cream milk, ice cream and cheese should be replaced with skimmed milk, unsweetened low fat yoghurt and low fat cheese. You could add some diced fruits to the yoghurt to 'jazz it up' or pour it over your cereal like muesli.

- White carbs like white bread, polished rice, cookies and so on, should be replaced with whole wheat versions. If you bake, you could add oatmeal to your cookies for a healthier option.

- Salt should be used very sparingly and the only way to do this is really re-training our taste buds to 'accept' less salt as tasty. Remember that you can use spices to 'jazz' up your food.

Over the weekends, some of us do quite a bit of cooking and I'm

PREPARING AND COOKING YOUR VEGGIES

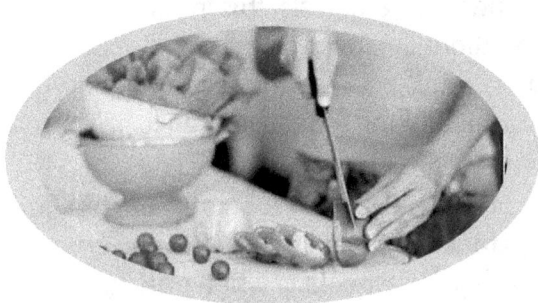

hoping, praying and keeping my fingers crossed that veggies will feature in this cooking spree.

Here are our top five tips for handling and cooking our vegetables in a healthy way.

When you buy vegetables in the market, buy them whole. Do not have them cut in the market. When you do this, you are exposing the very fragile water soluble vitamins in the vegetables to the air and denaturing them. And then you still have to wash them before use…this leads to bleeding out of the essential nutrients through the cut ends of the vegetables.

Then do not fry or over cook the vegetables. Simply lightly steam them in a pot with some spices as desired. Heat can actually break down and destroy fifteen to twenty percent of some of the vitamins in vegetables.

Research has shown that for vegetables like carrots, boiling is the best way of preserving the nutrients in carrots and sweet potatoes. Be sure to leave their skins on until after cooking. The anti-oxidant effects of tomatoes are also more pronounced after cooking.

Stir-frying. As the name suggests, this involves lightly greasing the pan with oil and continually stirring your thinly cut vegetables or cubed chicken breasts, emphasis on the words lightly greasing. For best results and shorter cooking time, use a really hot pan or wok.

Poaching. You can poach your vegetables in hot fluid…could be hot water, hot vegetable or meat stock. This preserves the nutrients and gives awesome flavour especially when poached in stock.

So, cook away…to your heart's content!

PREVENTION OF CROSS-CONTAMINATION OF FOOD

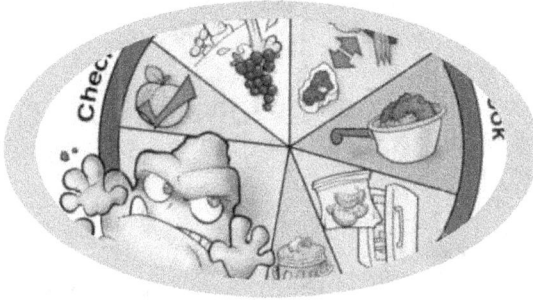

Harmful bacteria can pass from raw foods to other food products, some of which we even eat raw. These germs may not cause much harm to adults but could lead to very serious infections in children and other people with fragile immune systems.

Here are my top tips for preventing cross-contamination while shopping.

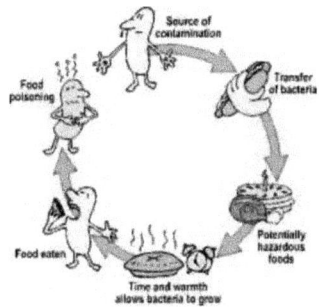

If you go to the open market, be sure to go with enough shopping bags. That way you can separate your raw meats/fish from your other foods.

If you shop in grocery stores, separate the foods in the shopping cart. You could use the shopping carts that have two baskets. Use one for your fish and meats and the other for your other food items.

When checking out your purchases at the grocery shops, ensure that the attendants pack these food stuffs in separate bags. In addition, keep dry foods separate from wet or refrigerated foods. This keeps the different foodstuff fresh until you get home and store them appropriately.

Maintain this separation in the car, bus or taxi that you will take home. It may be more convenient to pack everything in one bag, but I assure you it is not healthier.

Finally, before you start cooking, thoroughly wash your hands since you have handled money and loads of stuff which may have deposited myriads of germs on your hands.

If we keep our food safe from contamination from the time we buy them to the time we take them home, we have a better chance of ensuring they are fresh and deliver the right nutrients to us by the time we cook them.

FOOD HYGiENE

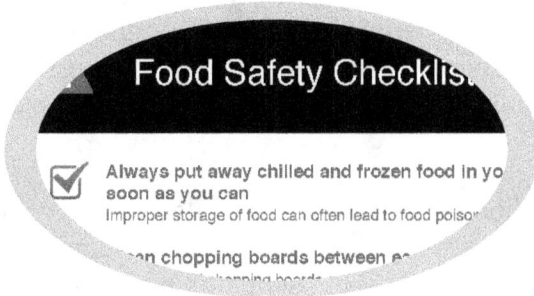

Food Safety Checklist

☑ Always put away chilled and frozen food in yo...
soon as you can
Improper storage of food can often lead to food poiso...

...on chopping boards between e...
...hopping boards...

What is food hygiene and how do you know you have been observing this in your kitchen? These are five things you need to know about food hygiene:

Eggs.   These are at the root of more than thirty percent of food poisoning cases. So get your children to stay off them. If you've got children like mine, it may not be as easy as it sounds especially when you've mixed up a batch of cakes and are trying to convince them that the batter they desperately want to lick off the bowl is not healthy! Ensure that egg dishes e.g. French toasts (when you choose to indulge) and custards are well cooked with no hint of raw eggs. The risk of salmonella infection is ever so real; so please be careful.

Chicken.   Poultry usually harbours the salmonella infection but because this meat is usually cooked before eating, it may not be a problem. However, cross contamination by using the same chopping board or work surface used to prepare chicken to prepare other foods could lead to salmonella infection. This is also the case if the chicken is stored in the fridge in direct contact with other foods. Use different work surfaces for raw meats and other foods and please separate from other foods when storing in the freezer.

Raw or slightly cooked fish.   All you sushi lovers, please pay attention. Worms in raw fish can survive in the intestines of man and cause infections; thus fish has to be properly cooked.

Appropriate cooking methods include grilling and poaching...you know, the way most people fry their fish until it sounds and feels like plantain chips when you're eating it? Well, that certainly will destroy any worm in the fish but is not healthy for you. Sounds like you can't win, yeah? 😵

Raw or partially cooked meat. Provided meat is not minced; any surface contamination of the meat is easily eliminated by cooking. However, minced meat requires that the meat be cooked thoroughly all the way through. Lovers of tartar which are raw meat dishes should be especially wary. Wooden chopping boards are discouraged as grooves formed on them while cutting items, form rich reservoirs for germs.

Fruits and vegetables are not common sources of food contamination but could get contaminated if prepared on a contaminated surface or if not in optimal quality when eaten. For these reasons you need to be careful.

Please make sure you obey the cardinal rules of hygiene in the kitchen as in every other part of your life. We must not forget to wash our hands thoroughly before we start cooking too. The saying that 'germs no dey kill African man,' is totally obsolete.

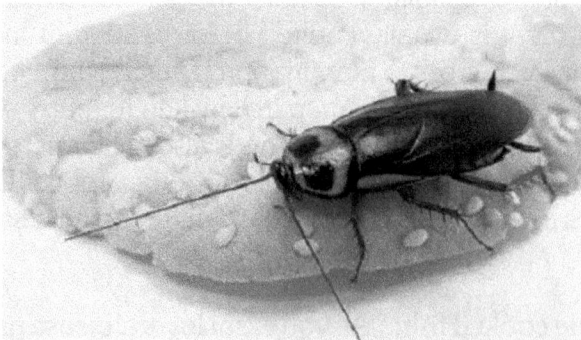

Q: There are germs inside raw vegetables. Sometimes, washing alone won't kill the germs. What do we do?

A: Truth is, there are germs all around us and potentially, in other foods we eat. But that doesn't mean that we should stop eating,

right? 🐝 We just need to figure out safe ways of preparing them and getting rid of germs that may be on their surface.

For green leafy veggies, buy them whole from the market. When you're ready to use them, pick the leaves and then soak in a bowl of water that has salt or food-safe disinfectant in it, for about five minutes. Swish the bowl around to ensure that all the sand settles to the bottom, then pick out the veggies carefully and rinse in clean water.

The same applies to other veggies too. For carrots and potatoes; buy them, scrub and then boil. If you wish to eat the carrots raw, just scrub and eat. For potatoes; scrub and boil before peeling.

With this, you should be home free! 😊

Q: Should we re-use oils that have been used for frying?

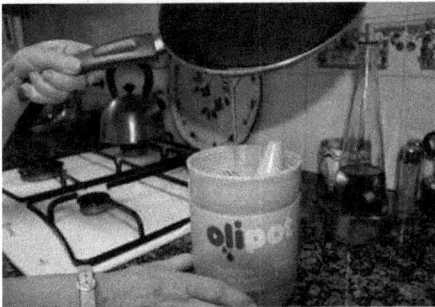

A: This is a very important question. How do we tell a woman who has used a whole pot of oil to fry akara (bean cakes) to pour all that oil away afterwards? In these tough economic times? The truth is, even if she wanted to do that for her health, the economic imperatives make it impossible! Do you know how much that oil cost?

Okay, so what can we do?

Re-using oil can be done safely, but you would need to determine if the oil has a high smoking point. 😊

Smoking point, simply put, is the heating point at which the oil begins to smoke.

From the definition above, we can deduce that oil that has reached its smoking point is not good for use anymore. In fact, you can consider smoking point to be that point at which oil goes from good to bad! At that point, the oil breaks down and forms free radicals that can cause cancer. Oils like peanut (groundnut) and Soya oils have high smoking points and do not break down easily.

Cooking oil is generally re-usable provided it doesn't get to its smoking point, foam, change colour or develop a funny smell.

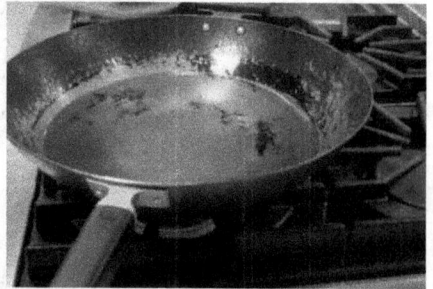

To store the oil, let it cool, strain out all the food debris and then put in jars (glass, preferably) and refrigerate or freeze and use within one month. If food debris is left in the oil, it forms a rich culture medium for micro-organisms that can cause food poisoning to grow.

Finally, as much as is practicable, try not to add salt to the food you wish to fry as salt lowers the smoking point of oils. And, by the way, what's with all the frying? …Grill, bake or roast.

Q: Is it good to store our cooked food in the refrigerator?

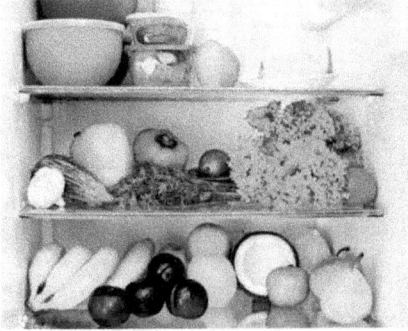

A: First of all, you have to be sure that the food you intend to store is good quality. We, oftentimes, have the impression that the fridge has some magical properties and so, if we put bad food in the fridge, it magically becomes good…or perhaps, if it was about to go bad, then the process of decay is halted. But this is not true. The fridge preserves the quality of what you have put in it and slows down the growth of germs that can cause the food to spoil. Please note the words 'slow down.' The process is delayed and not completely stopped, which is the reason why it's always a great idea to eat up food in the fridge within two to three days. The freezer can preserve food for much longer though, so if it's possible to freeze, please do.

Once food has been cooked, and you want to refrigerate or freeze, be sure to do so within two hours of preparation (by which time the food would have cooled) to prevent germs from taking residence. 😀

Other general tips to remember when storing foods in the fridge: Make sure the temperature of the unit is maintained at less than 5°C.

Clean your fridge often to guarantee that you're not actively growing germs in them. 😀

Be sure that all foods stored in the fridge or freezer are at least at room temperature before placing in the refrigerator. Storing hot foods straight in the fridge increases its temperature and encourages the growth of micro-organisms.

Store foods that go bad easily towards the back of the fridge where it's cooler e.g. milk and other dairy foods.

If your food is over-packed, that's also a problem as the cool air will not be able to circulate to keep things, nice, cool and fresh.

Once you have opened a can of food, take the food out of the can before storing in the fridge. If not, the food may get contaminated with the metal. Pour out the food into your storage containers and then place in the fridge.

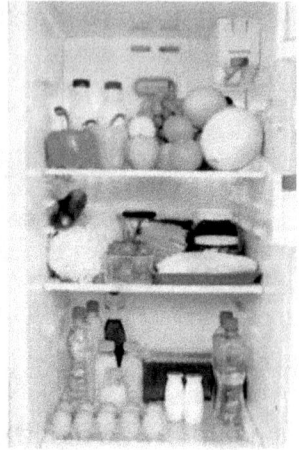

De-frost food completely before cooking and if you're in a hurry to use the meat immediately, defrost in the micro-wave. Then make sure, the food is cooked evenly all the way through.

If you have cause to store chicken or other meat in your fridge (like when marinating, i.e. mixed with spices to season it), it is important for it not to make contact with other food items. Store them in the bottom part of the fridge away from other foods to ensure that fluids from them don't drip onto other foods. And try not to store cooked meat together with raw meat to prevent the transfer of germs.

This is enough to get you thinking now, right?

Q: It has been noted that when vegetables are not properly cooked, there is a tendency of contracting some diseases like E. coli. What is the best way of cooking your vegetable?

A: It is not the improper cooking of the vegetables that pre-disposes a person to E. Coli infection, it is the preparation of the vegetables ab initio. Buy your vegetables whole from the market. 'For green leafy vegetables, pick the leaves and then soak and swish around in water that has some food safe sterilizing fluid or salt in it for a few minutes. Swishing helps the sand settle to the bottom and the food-safe sterilizing fluid 'sterilizes' the vegetables. Once this process is completed, it's ready for eating (like cabbage, lettuce, eggplant leaves or Swiss chard) or ready to be cut or cooked (spinach or Ugu leaves).

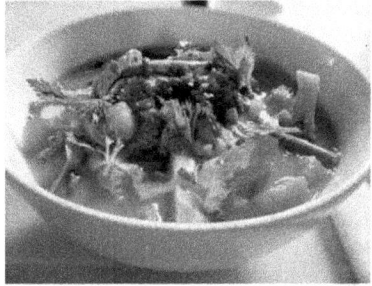

When cooking, try to minimize the amount of time food is exposed to heat, especially for green leafy veggies. You can stir fry (add a little oil to the pan and keep stirring the veggies to cook them in the oil), braise (add a little water and cook) or just wilt them. I prefer the latter, and I just add some onions, pepper and some seasoning to it, stir it around for a bit (two to three minutes) and it's good to go.

Part 4

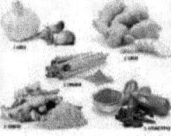

YOUR FOOD AND CANCER

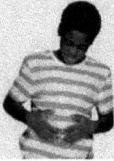

CONSTIPATION, BLOATING AND MORE

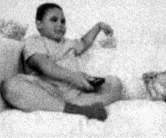

SNACKING

YOUR FOOD AND CANCER

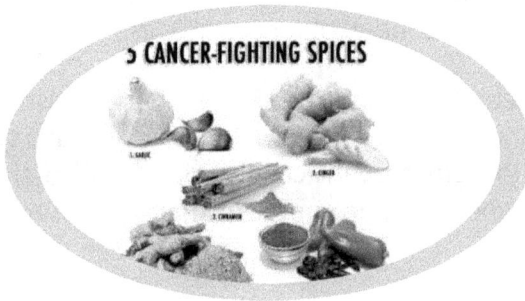

Our diet plays a huge role in our health...I'm sure I've said that, perhaps a gazillion times only. 😃 But, if ever you needed a reason to eat right, here it is. Some food tips to help you fight cancer:

Reduce your consumption of red meat and animal fat

Studies have shown that a diet high in animal fat increases the risk for several types of cancer. Poultry and fish contain less fat than red meat and so increasing these in your diet while reducing the red meat may help to prevent cancer. A diet high in fat also is a major cause of obesity, which is a risk factor for many types of cancer.

Reduce Your Alcohol Intake

Drinking excessive amounts of alcohol have been implicated as a risk factor for many types of cancer. Studies suggest that men who consume two alcoholic drinks per day and women who have one alcoholic drink per day increase their risk factors significantly for certain types of cancer. Remember that these are the generally 'approved' or 'recommended' limits of alcohol for men and women daily...spend a moment and just reflect on that.

Eat Your Fruits and Veggies

A diet rich in fruits and vegetables greatly reduces your risk of developing cancer and many other conditions.

Fruits and vegetables contain antioxidants, which help repair our damaged cells. Green, orange and yellow fruits and vegetables are your best bet to help prevent cancer. Studies also show that dark fruits, like blueberries and grapes, may also have anti-cancer properties.

Cruciferous vegetables such as cabbage, broccoli and cauliflower are especially useful in preventing cancer, according to numerous studies.

Avoid Smoking and Exposure to Smoke: Smoking has been implicated in not only lung cancer, but many other types of cancer. It is the most significant cancer risk factor that we can reduce by quitting or never starting.

Practice Safe Sex

Unsafe sex has been associated with cervical cancer. It can lead to infection with the human papilloma virus (HPV), which can cause cancer of the cervix and is a risk factor for other types of cancer. HPV is a common sexually transmitted infection that is spread through sexual, skin-to-skin contact. There is a vaccine to prevent this cancer now. Please ask your doctor. HIV/AIDS is also associated with some types of cancers. Get screened regularly.

Q: What functions do ginger and garlic serve in our bodies?

A: These are two great food seasonings. For people who use a lot of salt ordinarily, using these seasonings help to put the zing back in your food…they add a little something extra, such that you don't miss the salt that much. But, they are also healthy and good for you

Garlic: Yes, I know it gives you stinky breath but it is amazingly super healthy!

Funny...but it could very well be the sulphur-compounds causing that odour that also stop cancer-causing substances from forming in your body, speeds-up DNA repair, and kills cancer cells.

TOP 5 CANCER-CAUSING FOODS

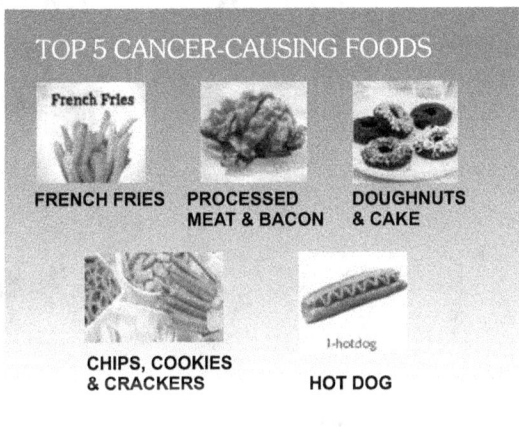

French Fries

FRENCH FRIES   PROCESSED   DOUGHNUTS
           MEAT & BACON   & CAKE

CHIPS, COOKIES
& CRACKERS   HOT DOG

1-hotdog

Garlic also battles bacteria, including **Helicobacter pylori** (the one connected to some ulcers and stomach cancer), and it reduces the risk of colon cancer.

To get the most benefit, peel and chop the cloves and let them sit fifteen to twenty minutes before cooking. That activates enzymes and releases the sulfur-containing compounds that have the most protective effect.

Ginger: When you chew ginger, gingerols come out and are helpful in preventing nausea and high blood pressure.

CONSTiPATiON, BLOATiNG AND MORE

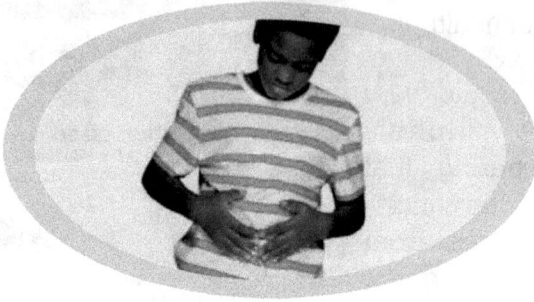

Have you ever been embarrassed by a growling stomach, a burp that came from nowhere or just that feeling of 'gassiness' (I'm not even sure this is a real word!). Well, you're not alone. Millions, the world over have also experienced this.

'Excess gas' is produced in the body when we swallow it or when our body produces it, as a result of what we have eaten. We are more likely to swallow air when we eat very fast, when we chew gum, drink through a straw or suck on hard candies. Certain foods cause our bodies to also produce gas. For example, beans, whole wheat grains, carbonated drinks and fruits like apples. These are mainly healthy foods (minus the carbonated drinks) and so we are not about to ask you to stop eating them. What you can do since you have this problem is to reduce the amounts of these foods that you eat.

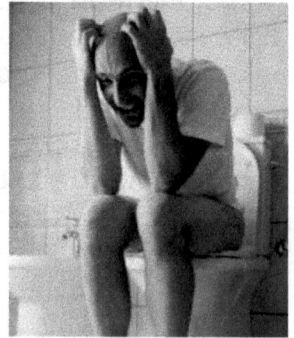

You could keep a food diary to identify the specific items that cause this problem for you and then, reduce those.

Q: What is the cause of constipation and how can it be prevented?

A: Constipation occurs when faeces passes too slowly down the digestive tract causing the stool to become hard and brittle. It leads to a situation where a person has less than three bowel movements per week. The classic symptoms are straining to pass stool, having the feeling of incomplete emptying after a poo and sometimes having to press down on your abdomen to **aid bowel movement in the toilet.** Sometimes, constipated people also insert a finger into their rectum to help the process along.

Constipation becomes chronic when it persists for weeks on end and it may be due to blockages in the rectum or as a result of diseases like Diabetes Mellitus. They could also be due to issues like not drinking enough water, not eating enough fibre in our meals and living a sedentary lifestyle. Being a woman and getting older also pre-disposes one to more episodes of constipation.

Prevention is focused on ensuring that you have enough fibre in your diet (fruits, vegetables, and whole grain), getting at least thirty minutes of exercise daily and drinking at least eight glasses of water daily. When you have the urge to poo, try not to delay it for too long. Go and take your time to do your business! 😆

Q: I have noticed that some people hardly chew their food before swallowing. Can this cause problems?

A: Okay, this brings up visions of people who literally inhale their food! You know those ones who are already done eating when people are still trying to get the first mouthful in. 😶

Well, yes this is a problem. In the first instance, hardly chewing your food means that you are eating it way too fast. One of the problems associated with this is that the person is likely to swallow a lot of air leading to a feeling of being bloated. Then, eating too fast too could lead to a situation where your stomach does not have enough time to communicate to your brain that you are full. So, you're probably already stuffed before you stop eating. This is a bad idea when we are thinking up ways to practice portion control.

Food that is not chewed properly is also much more difficult for the digestive enzymes in the stomach and even saliva to act on. Chewing your food properly to a watery paste before swallowing helps saliva and digestive juices act on it, thus, you get the benefit of all the nutrients in the food you have eaten.

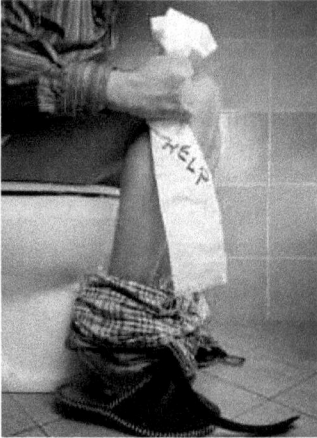

To make sure you're not guilty of this, take small bites of your food, chew slowly and intentionally, swallow the food in your mouth before you put more in. So, make a conscious effort today to eat slower. For obese people, it may not solve all weight loss problems (as other factors could be involved in their not feeling satisfied often), but it's a step in the right direction.

SNACKiNG

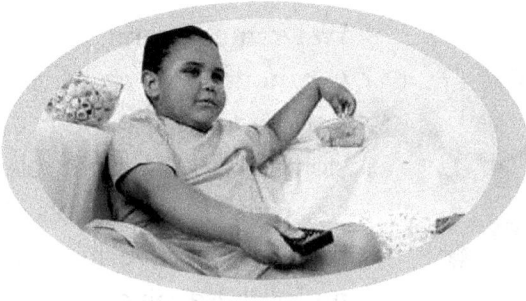

Do you find yourself getting hungry around 3.00pm…even if you've had lunch? Do you usually give in and get a doughnut or meat pie or take a soft drink perhaps? Well, none of those things are part of a healthy diet and indeed could cause more problems than the one they are trying to solve.

Healthier options to chew on at that time (or to use as snacks at any time, really) are nuts. Try a mix of different nuts like peanuts or groundnuts, almonds and cashew nuts…you could even throw in some currants. Remember that though nuts contain heart healthy oils, a little goes a long way. So stick to a handful, only. Avocado pears and fruit slices are also a great treat but try to cut up and refrigerate your own fruit slices or buy from a vendor you can trust. The type prepared by fruit sellers on the street usually sit out there baking in the sun for a long time before it's bought.

I am going to give you practical examples of fruits and vegetables in our environment that can take the edge off your hunger and still keep you healthy. Ever heard the saying, 'An apple a day keeps the doctor away'? Well, it is true. Eat them raw and include them in smoothies. Same goes for bananas, mangos, oranges and carrots.

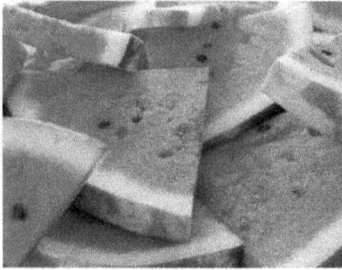

Water melon and pineapples are also very nourishing, and their health benefits are best experienced on an empty stomach. Blue berries, blackberries and strawberries contain lots of anti-oxidants that are effective in preventing cancer and all these can be eaten on their own or added to smoothies.

Smoothies are fruit juices extracted in a smoothie-maker...almost like blending the fruits. The smoothie-maker goes a step further by removing the pulp so that you are left with a pure fruit juice. Traditionally, yoghurts are added but be sure that they are the low fat and no-added sugar variety. To be extra certain you are not being fed 'hidden' sugars, you could make yours (a cup of milk to 4 cups of warm water. Leave in an airtight container overnight. Add a little amount of readymade yoghurt – unsweetened – to this and then refrigerate).

These fruits and vegetables also come packed with vitamins, minerals and lots of other benefits:

Apples are known to be anti-cancer health promoters and also helpful in reducing blood pressure.

Bananas help to keep hunger pangs away as they bring about a slow release of energy.

Mangoes mop-up free radicals and stimulate the immune system. (By the way, free radicals are produced by the body as part of the natural process of converting food to energy; they can also be extracted from the air and generated by the sun's action on skin and eyes. These toxic substances can start off a domino-like chain reaction leading to malfunctioning and dead cells and ultimately, a lot of diseases in the body). I'm sure you need a breather here just to digest this ☺

Take a deep breath…

Oranges aid the destruction of free radicals (again) that cause skin aging.Carrots promote healthy skin and eyes. Watermelon is refreshing and helps reduce blood pressure. Pineapples aid digestion and aid in dissolving mucus. Blueberries, blackberries and strawberries destroy free radicals (yet again!) and slow down the signs of aging.

Talking about smoothies, do you know you can live on a diet of raw fruits and vegetables made into smoothies for days? Okay, just before you decide on the particular (unpleasant) name you want to call me, perhaps starting off with a day and then graduating to three days is a better idea.

Away with the face that says 'Yuck and all manners of eeew'. The smoothies do taste good and more importantly are good for you. You come away after three days feeling light and absolutely refreshed PLUS; you will see that tummy bulge reduce…bearing in mind that the quantum of reduction has to do with the initial size. The more the paunch (afo ukwu in Ibo or beer belly in ordinary parlance, the less visible the outward effect (but the inward cleansing and detoxification is constant). ☺

Fruits and veggies like celery, beetroot, apples, pineapples, black berries, blueberries, avocado pears, pumpkin leaves (ugu), lemon (with its rind), cucumber, ginger and carrots are some of the ingredients used in their raw state to make different smoothies for the three-day period. The vegetable, green (as known by us Okoros) or efo tete (as known by my Yoruba peeps) can also be added to the blend.

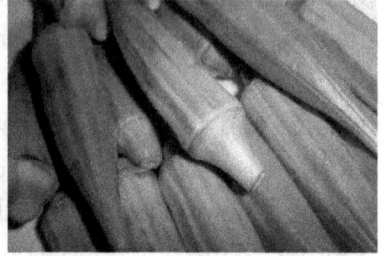

Check for these fruits and vegetables in the fruits and vegetable sections of major supermarkets. Truth is you can mix and match any of the ingredients. My favourite smoothie 'brew' is pineapple, watermelon, bananas and some mangoes when in season. The pineapples and watermelon go in the smoothie-maker. Then the smoothie (fruit blend) is added to the bananas and mango pulp in the blender, and it's all whizzed up….Scrumplicious!

For those with a sweet tooth, you can still take a teensy-weensy bit of chocolate. BUT, focus on the dark variety.

Lemon has vitamins and possesses cleansing properties. A slice of lemon in cold or hot water is a great energy booster and taking a cup of warm water with a lemon slice is a great way to start the day. A slice of lemon in cold water or blended in a smoothie-maker with beetroot and water added to it, is a healthy detoxifying brew for all times.

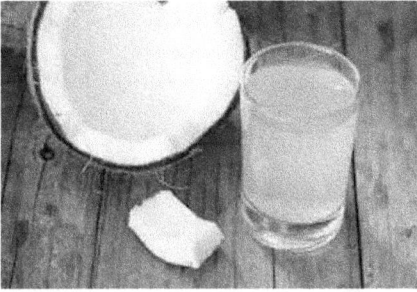

Coconut water is also a good way of preventing dehydration, and I have always been baffled by people who break the coconuts and pour away the water. As children growing up in my home, we devised all sorts of schemes to prevent the loss of any drop of the coconut water including using corkscrews at the bottom part that has three indentations and positioning it right over a cup. Those were the days (sigh)!

Green salads without all the fatty dressings are also great. Balsamic vinegar is better as salad dressing as it is derived from vines and rich in anti-oxidants. Be wary of the plastic-packed varieties of fruit and vegetable salad hawked by vendors which have good intentions at the root of it. But those fruits and veggies spend so much time baking in the sun that when they are eaten, they pose more of a health hazard than benefit! Avocado pears with their heart-healthy oils can be used as a spread on wheat bread sandwiches and also in salads.

Nuts, as I noted above, are also a good way to snack. Almonds, cashew nuts and pistachio nuts are good examples of nuts with fiber, protein and Omega 3 fatty acids (the good fatty acid). These nuts are available in all major supermarkets either as mixed nuts or one-nut packs. A small handful of peanuts (or groundnuts) will also not go amiss due to its high content of unsaturated fats and protein. Try to go for the unsalted and dry roasted varieties of all the nuts as opposed to the oil roasted ones. Walnuts are healthy and are pretty cheap when in season. They are called ukpa in Ibo and Asala or Awusa in Yoruba.

In fact, there is evidence that this could boost fertility in men. You are absolutely allowed to go nutty here.

Snack on mixed nuts: Especially in the mid-afternoon, this is a very effective pick-me-up that gives you a boost when your energy levels are waning. And they are also filled with heart healthy oils.

Do not wait too long between meals. This will lead to sugar levels falling too low, increase your cravings and make you over-indulge when you do get to eat.

Keep healthy snack options within reach in your fridge and cabinet. This should include lots of fruits as it makes it easier to pick healthier choices when snacking.

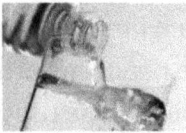

Drink water and often too. Sometimes, it is actually thirst that we feel and misread as hunger. Aim for at least 8 glasses of water a day and actually more if the weather is super-hot.

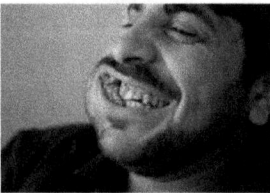

Chew slowly when you eat. Make a conscious effort to chew every bite and savour every single bit of it. . Since the stomach needs about fifteen minutes to get the signal that it is fed, this gives your tummy enough time to realize that it is actually full and reduces the amount of food you eventually eat. So don't just inhale your food; rather, enjoy every mouthful and give your stomach the chance to report 'I am full.'

No more excuses guys. On the go, at home… you have got healthy snacking options. Go for it.

More
QUESTIONS
And
Answers

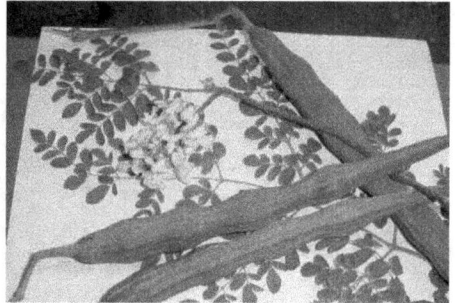
More
QUESTIONS
And
Answers

Q: Are Moringa seeds healthy and should we swallow Moringa seeds and leaves?

A: I have received so many questions about this Moringa that I decided to find out about it. Here's what I found out. It is touted to be a Miracle tree and a super food containing about ninety-two nutrients and about forty-six anti-oxidants. Every part of this plant is believed to be useful from the leaves, root, and fruits to the seeds. It is thought to cure myriads of diseases and prevent scores of others and is believed to be useful in purifying water, effective against bacteria and fungi, anti-hypertensive and cholesterol lowering activities, etc.

Some studies suggest that more work needs to be done to confirm its precise actions but one thing appears to be clear, there are clearly phytochemicals in the leaves that make the claims to curative and preventive care, factual.

I would also say that since it is a food supplement (even if it is a super food), be sure to get most of your nutrients from a healthy diet made up of other fruits and vegetables. Remember that supplements plug holes and are not supposed to be the mainstay of your diet. Also check out the contents and confirm that you are not allergic to any of the components before use.

Q: How should I break a fast?

A: Breaking a fast is usually not as easy as it seems. Since you haven't had a meal in a while, and it's suddenly time to eat, it's easy for you to pick anything you see and munch on it. Pretty open and shut, isn't it? But actually, it's not that simple.

For starters, during a fast, your digestive system takes a break. Therefore, it only makes sense to re-introduce your body to food gradually with easy to digest meals.

If you have ever tried to load your body with food immediately after a fast, you will recall the horrible cramps that followed as a result of trying to waken a sleeping digestive system too quickly.

Most people would break with citrus fruits like oranges, but their acidic content may be too much for your stomach to handle. However, easy-to-digest fruits like grapes, watermelons and apples are great options as they are readily absorbed while providing the body with needed energy and nutrients. Whether you choose to blend it into a juice or eat slices of them…it doesn't matter.

Remember that during your fast, given that you're on a calorie restrictive diet, go easy on the exercises and focus on stretching and gentle walks.

Q: Why is it that diabetics sweat a lot?

A: Everyone sweats when they have exerted themselves physically like after exercise, staying out on a hot day, staying in a poorly ventilated room or even when anxious. However, sweating in a cool room with no source of anxiety may mean that things are not

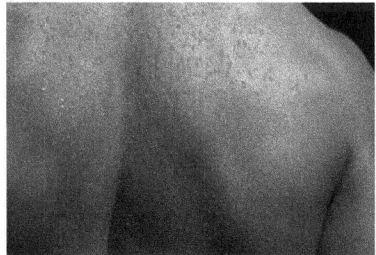

'A-okay.' This is usually typified by night-sweats which are not related to sleeping in a stuffy room.

Do diabetics sweat more than others? Yes and I'll tell you why. The high sugar level in Diabetes is thought to affect nerve function in several different ways. One of the ways is by affecting the nerves that control involuntary body functions (Diabetic Autonomic Neuropathy) like sweating, urinating, sexual arousal, etc. This can lead to increased or reduced activities of the organs involved. For instance:

If it affects the intestines, people experience diarrhoea or constipation.

If it affects the stomach, it can limit the ability of food to move through the digestive system causing bloating and vomiting.

If it affects the nerves that control erection when there is sexual arousal, it can lead to erectile dysfunction. However, the sexual desire is unaffected.

It can cause paralysis of the bladder such that the usual impulse to urinate when the bladder is full is lost. This leads to urine being stored for long periods in the bladder causing Urinary Tract Infections.

It can even blunt people's normal response to low blood sugar such that they no longer feel the warning signs and can't take preventive measures.

Diabetics, still as a result of nerve damage, either sweat a lot or don't even sweat when hot.

So, if you are diabetic or know anyone who is, blood sugar control is very important.

Q: Kindly enlighten me on the recommended quantity of water one is required to take each day. My concern is that after taking a glass of water, five minutes later, I go to bathroom. Is there something wrong with me?

A: Water is important for life and we use it for very important functions daily. Examples include taking a bath, washing clothes, washing dishes, cooking and of course, drinking. The water we drink is very critical for a lot of bodily functions like digestion, excretion (when we urinate, pass faeces and sweat), movement of nutrients all around the body, keeping your joints nice and supple, etc. If you also consider the fact that a healthy body contains about two-thirds, water, then it is clear that we can't joke with our water intake per day.

So how much should we drink every day? Though, there are recommended amounts, it really depends on your activity level (notice how much more water you appear to need after a hectic workout?), where you live (notice how much water you also seem to drink when you live or visit the tropics as opposed to when you live in or visit a temperate region?) and your health condition (for instance, people with Urinary Tract Infection need to drink some more water).

Generally, we are encouraged to drink eight 8-ounce glasses of fluid per day. This is approximately two litres of water each day. Honestly, though it breaks my heart to admit it any fluid counts.☺ For example, fruit juices and beverages could add to your recommended daily water intake but remember that these other fluid sources, other than water, may contain calories that you probably don't need. 😐

An easy way to check whether your body is getting enough water is to examine your urine colour. If it's dark yellow, you're probably not getting enough. If it's pale yellow in colour, you're doing well. 😊

200

If you don't like the taste of plain water, you can jazz it up with a slice of lemon or lime

When you first start trying to drink more water, you may observe an increase in your bathroom visits. This should stop after a short while. If it doesn't, please see your doctor. It may be an over-active bladder, a Urinary Tract Infection or some other illness.

Q: What is the effect of energy drinks and coffee on the body?

A: Hmm! Talking about coffee brings back memories of Medical School. I always used to love reading on my bed. Yep, you heard me. On my bed, surrounded by tomes of text books but just chilling and reading. This was my routine until it was time for my first major exam in Med-School…the second medical board exams! I felt that this was a special occasion which required a bit more from me. And so, I decided I was going to team up with a couple of my friends, go to class or the library and 'swot' till forever! Well, that was the plan. What eventually happened was a different story all together!

One of the first principles of 'swotting forever' is to ensure that you have a 'never-ending' supply of coffee. I had never been a coffee lover; so this was new territory! And so, I set off trying to brew my cuppa. I should have asked for advice from a veteran…I mean, that's common sense, isn't it? But no! I was convinced I knew exactly what needed to be done. And so I loaded the cup with instant coffee, added hot water, sugar and milk, and I was ready to face my medical tomes! Within minutes though, I realised something was terribly wrong! My tummy was rumbling, grumbling and roaring all at once! I raced into the toilet and spent the rest of the day there! There went my dream of swotting forever!

Moral of this story: Don't try to be like anyone else. If reading on your bed works for you, please go ahead and do just that. I learnt that the hard way! But, I digress…

Back to the question, energy drinks and coffee contain one important ingredient, caffeine. This is found in teas, chocolates and some sodas, too. Apart from the laxative effect it had on me, caffeine has other actions on the body:

- ○ Inability to sleep (I'm sure we all know that.

  That was the effect I was headed for and ended up with something else) 😝

- ○ Rapid heart beat
- ○ Irritability
- ○ Nervousness
- ○ Irritation of the bladder
- ○ High blood pressure and so on.

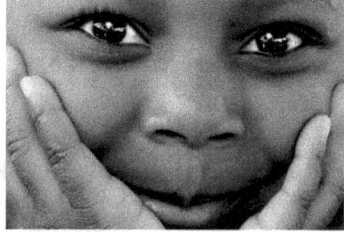

The recommended daily amount of caffeine is 400mg which is about the amount of coffee in two 8-ounce cups of coffee. These are the dainty cups of coffee and not the huge mug-like (Who-send-you-come?) cups that a lot of us favour. 😁

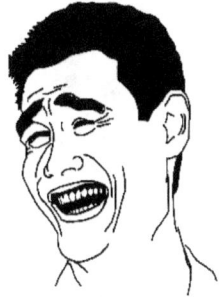

The energy drinks often contain huge amounts of caffeine and are used by people as a pick-me-up for different reasons. The thing is, if you haven't slept for three days and you're trying to complete that project by taking more energy drinks that will keep you awake, you will eventually pay for this…one way or the other. It is either the side-effects of caffeine take over or you do fall asleep! You can't cheat nature (forgive the cliché). Your body needs rest when it needs rest, and it will get it one way, or another!

So, if you must, one energy drink (about 500mls) once in a blue moon may not hurt you but it may be more constructive to try to pace your activities and not try to get everything done at once. Eat healthy and get some exercise (at least thirty minutes) daily. Mixing these drinks with alcohol and other recreational drugs makes it a more dangerous 'concoction.'

Please avoid energy drinks if you have been diagnosed with high blood pressure or you have a heart disease or at least speak to your doctor about it. Children and adolescents should stay off this. Pregnant women and breast feeding mothers should be especially careful.

Credits - Image Links

Pregancy

Cover (inner)	-	thedoctorschannels.com
Opening cover	-	healthyguts.net
Pregnant women	-	theguardian.com, page 1
Scanning	-	popsugar.com, page 3
Breast tenderlness	-	thealphaparent.com, page 7
Frequent urination	-	theasianparent.com, page 7
Morning sickness or nausea	-	diseasespictures.com, page 8
Crampy abdominal pain	-	blog.psibands.com, page 9
Pregnant woman eating	-	myhoustonmajic.com, page 10
Pregnant woman eating (2)	-	naturalbrownwoman.com, page 10
Big baby	-	fanpop.com, page 14
Diaperbag	-	overstock.com, page16
Hospital bag	-	seatlenewbornblog.com, page 17
Black pregnant couple	-	mommynoire.com, page 24
How to cope with my new wife	-	askmissa.com, page 29
Daddy or father	-	moeders.nu, page 23
Black couple	-	google.com, page 24
After birth	-	theblaze.com, page 25
Diaper change	-	intelligentnest.com, page 26
Immunization	-	dailypost.com, page 28
Immunization(2)	-	thelibertybeacon.com, page 28
Immunization(3)	-	fsg.org, page 28
Immunization(4)	-	humanosphere.org, page 29
Cord care	-	theparenting-magazine.com, page 30
Sitz bath	-	moondragon.org, page 30
Sitz bath kits	-	mountainside-medical.com, page 31
Baby cord	-	nezuqe.freehostingchamp.com, page 31
Mother and child	-	pinterest.com, page 32
My tummy after my baby	-	babycenter.com, page 38
Baby crying	-	practicingparents.com, page 40
Baby crying(2)	-	theguardian.com, page 40
Baby yawning	-	babymagz.com, page 41
Wet or dirty diaper	-	inthemommybusiness.com, page 42
Diapering 101	-	babymed.com, page 43
Diaper rash	-	dimomessentials.com, page 45
Planning an outing with baby	-	womenworld.org, page 46
wipes	-	thebluebottletree.com, page 46
Changing diaper	-	patheos.com, page 47

Diet Book